LOSE WHEAT
IN 4 WEEKS

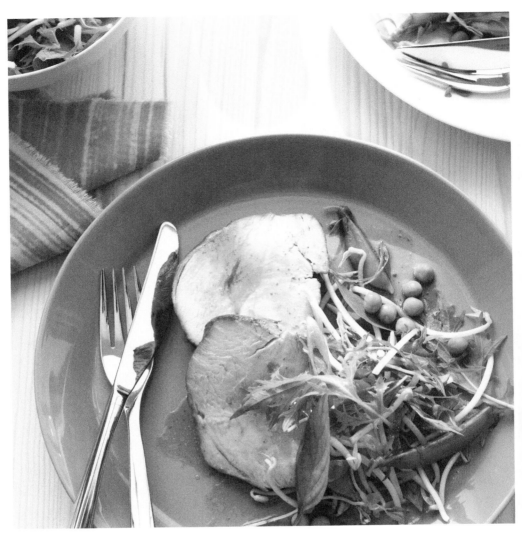

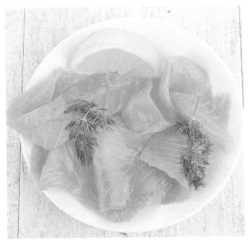

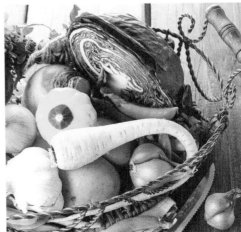

LOSE WHEAT
IN 4 WEEKS

AN EASY PLAN TO KICK GRAINS

SONOMA
PRESS

For general information on our other products and services or to obtain technical support, please contact our Customer Care Department within the U.S. at (866) 744-2665, or outside the U.S. at (510) 253-0500.

Sonoma Press publishes its books in a variety of electronic and print formats. Some content that appears in print may not be available in electronic books, and vice versa.

TRADEMARKS: Sonoma Press and the Sonoma Press logo are trademarks or registered trademarks of Callisto Media Inc. and/or its affiliates, in the United States and other countries, and may not be used without written permission. All other trademarks are the property of their respective owners. Sonoma Press is not associated with any product or vendor mentioned in this book.

Photo credits: ISTL/Stockfood, p. ii (top); Bernhard Winkelmann/Stockfood, p. vi; Eising Studio–Food Photo & Video/Stockfood, p. ix (bottom right); Eising Studio–Food Photo & Video/Stockfood, p. x; Michael Wissing/Stockfood, p. 10; Louis Hiemstra/Getty Images, p. 20; Anthony Lanneretonne/Stockfood, p. (top); Eising Studio–Food Photo & Video/Stockfood, p. 34; Miki Duisterhof/Stockfood, p. 50; Charles Schiller Photography/Stockfood, p. 55; Maya Visnyei/Stockfood, p. 61; Alan Richardson/Stockfood, p. 67; Leigh Beisch/Stockfood, p. 72; Spyros Bourboulis/Stockfood, p. 89; House & Leisure/Stockfood, p. 94; Sporrer/Skowronek/Stockfood, p. 101; Valerie Janssen/Stockfood, p. 108; Tina Rupp/Stockfood, p. 115; és-cuisine/Stockfood, p. 118; Eising Studio–Food Photo & Video/Stockfood, p. 123; Leigh Beisch/Stockfood, p. 127; Sven Benjamins/Stockfood, p. 132; Roger Stowell/Stockfood, p. 136; Oliver Brachat/Stockfood, p. 141; Snowflake Studios Inc./Stockfood, p. 147; Sarah Coghill/Stockfood, p. 152; Jennifer Martine/Stockfood, p. 157; David Loftus/Stockfood, p. 160; Charles Schiller Photography/Stockfood, p. 164; Keller & Keller Photography/Stockfood, p. 169; Maja Smend/Stockfood, p. 172; Jalag-Syndication/Wolfgang Schardt/Stockfood, p. 181; Gräfe & Unzer Verlag/Jörn Rynio/Stockfood, p. 184; Debi Treloar/Stockfood, p. 189; Boguslaw Bialy/Stockfood, p. 194; Rose Hodges/Stockfood, p. 198; Louise Lister/Stockfood, p. 204; Mans Jensen/Stockfood, p. 211; Keller & Keller Photography/Stockfood, p. 218; Chris Meier/Stockfood, p. 225; Jo Kirchherr/Stockfood, p. 229; Tina Rupp/Stockfood, p. 232; Great Stock!/Stockfood, p. 238; Snowflake Studios Inc./Stockfood, p. 242; Adrian Lawrence/Stockfood, p. 249; Harry Bischof/Stockfood, p. 259; Louise Lister/Stockfood, p. 264; Clinton Hussey/Stockfood, p. 273; Bianca Brandon-Cox/Stockfood, p. 290; Food and Drink Photos/Food Image Collection/Stockfood, p. 295; Rob Fiocca Photography/Stockfood, p. 296. All other photographs www.shutterstock.com.

ISBN: Print 978-0-9895586-7-9

Contents

Introduction

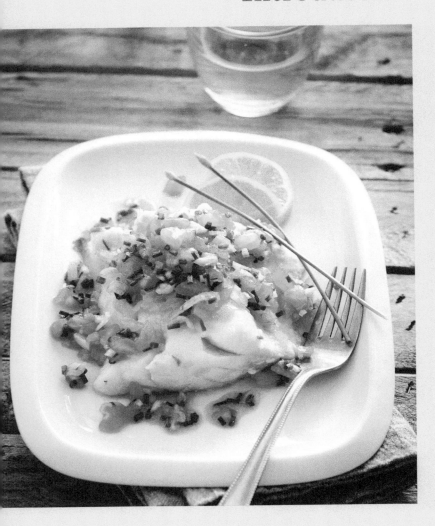

R eady to experience the health benefits of going grain-free without forfeiting flavor? You're in luck. *Lose Wheat in 4 Weeks* is packed with easy grain-free recipes that will appeal to your taste buds and work for your budget and busy schedule. This cookbook provides all the recipes you need to get started, with shopping lists and day-by-day menu suggestions.

Grains are defined as the seeds of plants (such as wheat, corn, and millet) that are used for food. They are found in many of the foods we eat—pasta, bread, cakes, cereals, and snack foods. Grains are often hidden in foods that you may think are grain-free, such as soy products, protein powders, flavored teas, and baking powder. You can bet that the vegetable burgers you bought have some sort of grain thickener in them. The list goes on and on.

But giving up grain is well worth the effort. Switching to a grain-free diet may help individuals who struggle with their weight, high blood sugar, chronic inflammation, digestive disorders, and various neurological disorders. If you are tired of yo-yoing between feeling great at your ideal weight and feeling sluggish, heavy, and overweight, or if you have been looking for a dietary approach to combating various chronic conditions, or if you are ready to feel more energetic and focused every day, then it's time to get into the kitchen and start cooking.

Every recipe in *Lose Wheat in 4 Weeks* has just a handful of supermarket-friendly ingredients and takes 45 minutes or less to cook, leaving you more time to sit down and enjoy a home-cooked meal. You'll begin with the fastest recipes for familiar favorites, each with 5 to 10 minutes of prep time. As the weeks progress, the recipes become a bit more sophisticated, and you'll improve your cooking skills, which will help keep you motivated as you progress through your grain-free detox. By the end of the four-week program, you can expect even better blood sugar control, fewer hunger pangs and cravings between meals, improved sleep, higher energy levels throughout the day, and most importantly, significant and sustained weight loss. In other words, you'll be able to lose the pounds and keep them off—which is something everyone wants.

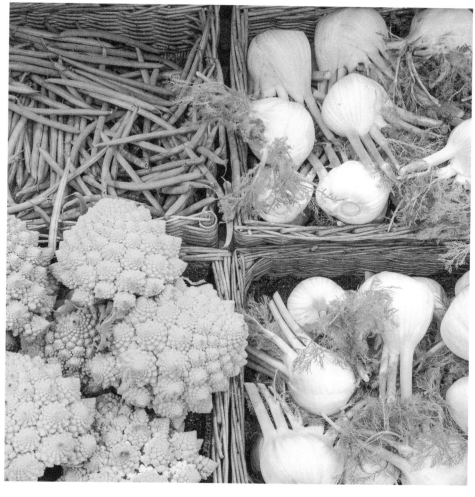

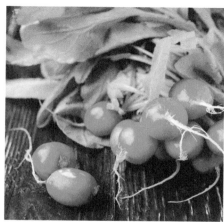

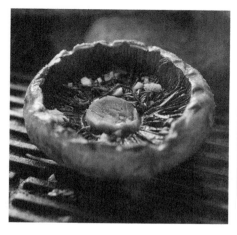

CHAPTER 1

Why Go Grain-Free?

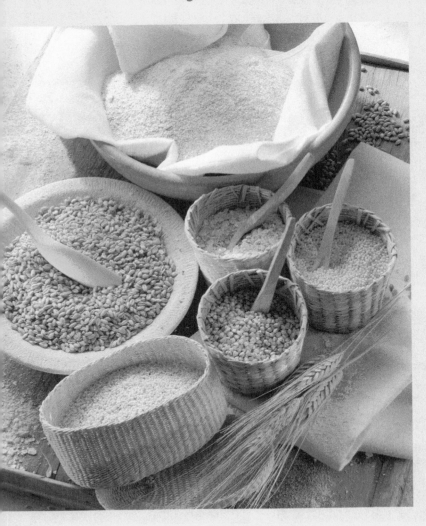

Walking into your neighborhood bookstore, you see a display of diet cookbooks and think, "Another diet? No, thank you." After all, anyone with a healthy level of skepticism knows that diet trends come and go almost as frequently as fashion fads and Hollywood careers. But the grain-free diet seems to be different. It has already captured the minds of many Americans, as seen by the popularity of New York Times best sellers Wheat Belly and Grain Brain and the Paleo and Keto diets. Why?

These lifestyle-changing diets turn the conventional wisdom of well-respected establishments like the USDA, American Diabetes Association, American Heart Association, and the Academy of Nutrition and Dietetics on their heads. Those dietary programs encourage you to eat plenty of whole grains and to minimize cholesterol and fat intake. But rather than making you slimmer and healthier, whole grains could be doing the exact opposite: making you fatter and sicker.

Does this sound crazy? It probably does at first glance. But a run through the latest scientific studies leaves even the most skeptical people wondering if everything they've ever been told in the past 30 years about healthy eating has been wrong.

One day, people may look back and realize that encouraging people to eat 6 to 11 servings of grains a day is like saying that margarine loaded with unhealthy trans-fats is healthier than butter.

The Effects of Eating Grains

So, how exactly does eating whole grains (or any grains for that matter) make you sick?

Let's start with wheat. Wheat, according to William Davis, MD, author of Wheat Belly, "is the dominant source of gluten protein in the human diet. . . . Wheat consumption overshadows consumption of other gluten-containing grains by more than a hundred to one." Wheat is second only to corn in terms of acreage, and Davis says, "It is, by a long stretch, among the most consumed grains on earth, constituting 20 percent of all calories consumed."

Modern wheat is mostly composed of a type of carbohydrate that is readily digested and converted into blood sugar. It's not surprising then that it has a particularly adverse effect on blood sugar levels, causing them to increase far more than they would with just about any other source of carbohydrates. Whether you're eating slices of whole-grain organic bread or refined white bread, it makes no difference. A 2002 study in the *American Journal of Clinical Nutrition* demonstrated that when participants consumed whole-kernel rye bread and whole-wheat pasta, their bodies had the same glucose response as they did after consuming white bread made from white wheat flour. According to *Wheat Belly*, a 1981 University of Toronto study found that the glycemic index of whole-grain bread was higher than that of table sugar (72 versus 59). "Advice to consume more healthy whole grains therefore causes increased consumption of . . . a form of carbohydrate that, for all practical purposes, is little different, and in some ways worse, than dipping your spoon into the sugar bowl," says Dr. Davis.

Elevated blood sugar levels lead to elevated insulin levels, and ultimately, the conversion of excess sugar into fat, which mostly settles around the abdomen, the most dangerous kind. Abdominal fat is different from fat located anywhere else on the body—Dr. Davis considers

WHAT IS THE GLYCEMIC INDEX?

The glycemic index (GI) is a measure of how much a particular food or ingredient increases blood sugar within a 90- to 120-minute window, relative to pure glucose, which has a score of 100. A food which scores above 100 increases blood sugar more than glucose, and a food which scores below 100 increases blood sugar less than glucose. A score of 0 indicates that the ingredient has no impact on blood sugar.

AN OVERVIEW OF GRAIN-FREE DIETS

With all of the grain-free diets out there, it can be difficult to keep them straight. Here's a list of some of the most popular ones.

Wheat Belly diet: Dr. Davis's diet plan calls for the unlimited consumption of all vegetables, raw nuts and seeds, healthy oils, fresh animal-based protein, cheese (except for blue cheese, which is exposed to bread mold), non-sugary condiments, avocados, olives, coconut, spices, and cocoa. He advises that dieters consume non-cheese dairy such as milk, yogurt, and butter in limited quantities and also limit fruit consumption. Berries are preferable to other kinds of fruit because of their higher acid and lower sugar content. Fruit juices and gluten-free grains like buckwheat and rice, legumes, and soy products are permissible in small quantities. Cured meats, wheat products, refined polyunsaturated oils such as corn oil, and processed foods are to be avoided.

Paleo diet: Often referred to as the "caveman diet," the Paleolithic diet is similar to the *Wheat Belly* diet except that it does not allow for consuming any cereal grains, dairy, legumes, or potatoes. The Paleo diet does allow for unlimited consumption of fruit. It also calls for meats that are grass-fed rather than grain-fed. Of the four diets discussed here, it is the only true grain-free diet.

Keto diet: Short for the "ketogenic diet," this is the most extreme of all the diets outlined here. According to Dr. Perlmutter, "A purely ketogenic diet is one that derives 80 to 90 percent of calories from fat, and the rest from carbohydrate and protein." While not completely grain-free, those who follow the diet eliminate grains if they are adhering strictly to the guidelines. The theory is that by minimizing carbohydrate intake, the body will be forced to go into a ketotic state, meaning the brain is forced to turn to body fat as a fuel source. Since the brain is a major user of the body's energy—even at rest, the brain consumes 22 percent—this can result in significant weight loss.

Grain Brain diet: Dr. Perlmutter's diet is similar to the *Wheat Belly* diet, except that it incorporates elements of the Keto diet. Followers reduce their intake of carbohydrates to just 30 to 40 grams a day for the first month, followed by a daily maximum of just 60 grams. It also calls for increased cholesterol and fat consumption. Perlmutter's argument is that the brain runs best when given a steady supply of fat. And for those worried that eating fat will make them fat, according to a 2000 study published in the *American Journal of Clinical Nutrition*, fat consumption may actually turn off the body's own factory for making triglycerides, or fat molecules. Dr. Perlmutter argues that the same goes for cholesterol. He says, "Eating high-cholesterol foods has no impact on our actual cholesterol levels, and the alleged correlation between higher cholesterol and higher cardiac risk is an absolute fallacy."

it a separate gland, and the more it grows, the more it contributes to a never-ending cycle of greater insulin resistance, inflammation, and elevated triglyceride and "bad cholesterol" (small LDL) levels in the blood. Each of these, in turn, causes another set of health conditions.

Over time, untreated insulin resistance results in diabetes. According to the American Diabetes Association, 29.1 million American children and adults are diabetic, and another 86 million age 20 and older are pre-diabetic. Most alarming, diabetes outpaces any other disease in America in terms of annual growth. Diabetes often leads to further complications such as vision and circulatory problems, kidney failure, and nerve damage.

Moreover, according to Dr. Davis, wheat is chemically addictive. Consumption of wheat causes the body to want more food, leading to increased calorie consumption and compounding the problem.

What's the solution? Simple: Lose the wheat, along with the weight.

Diabetes is not the only chronic disease that Dr. Davis links to wheat consumption, though. He says the inflammation caused by the aforementioned abdominal fat is a precursor to hypertension, heart disease, colon cancer, dementia, and rheumatoid arthritis. The accumulation of small LDL particles in the walls of arteries also contributes to heart attacks, and the consumption of wheat causes those particles to oxidize, compounding their effect.

He also asserts that the consumption of wheat, when not balanced sufficiently with vegetable intake, can throw off the delicate pH balance

WHAT IS INSULIN RESISTANCE?

Insulin is a hormone that is manufactured and released by the pancreas in response to the intake of sugar. It allows sugar to enter the body's cells. An increase in blood sugar levels requires more insulin to be released to keep the process going, but sustained levels of high blood sugar can result in cells becoming progressively less sensitive to insulin. This requires the pancreas to produce even more insulin in response, and a vicious cycle results—repeated cycles of high blood sugar will eventually cause the pancreas to tire out, which leads to diabetes.

of blood and turn it acidic, leading eventually to bone loss and osteoporosis. And, the consumption of wheat results in increased levels of a compound that promotes premature aging.

The brain is also vulnerable to the effects of wheat (and other grains), according to Dr. Perlmutter, author of *Grain Brain*. He argues that "the shift in our diet that has occurred over the past century—from high-fat, low-carb to today's low-fat, high-carb diet, fundamentally consisting of grains and other damaging carbohydrates—is the origin of many of our modern scourges linked to the brain, including chronic headaches, insomnia, anxiety, depression, epilepsy, movement disorders, schizophrenia, ADHD, and those senior moments that quite likely herald serious cognitive decline." To stave off these chronic conditions of the brain, he proposes a carbohydrate-restricted diet (see page 3) based on the principles of the Keto diet.

The elimination of wheat and other grains is not novel for some groups of people. For people who follow the Paleo diet, avoiding grains is a part of everyday life. For the millions who suffer from celiac disease, eliminating wheat, rye, barley, triticale and other sources of gluten, the protein that promotes inflammation and its associated health problems, is the cornerstone of their treatment. And for people suffering from irritable bowel syndrome and other digestive disorders, avoiding wheat, rye, barley, and spelt can relieve their digestive distress significantly. In addition, a growing number of Americans are discovering that they have gluten allergies or wheat sensitivities; for them, going wheat-free can lead to a much healthier and more comfortable life.

There are many theories as to why wheat and other grains today can cause so many health problems. In the case of wheat, Davis blames the aggressive hybridization that has taken place over the past century or so in the name of increasing crop yields and disease resistance. As a result, wheat today is far different from the wild einkorn that our ancestors originally planted thousands of years ago. Today, there are over 25,000 varieties of wheat, all with subtly different biochemical properties and dozens of varieties of gluten, with health effects that are just now starting to be realized.

Although *Lose Wheat in 4 Weeks* offers a meal plan and recipes for a 100 percent grain-free diet, it is recommended that readers, especially those with pre-existing conditions, talk with their doctors before pursuing any serious changes to their diet.

The Five Essential Guidelines for a Grain-Free Diet

1. **Eat whole foods**. If you replace grains with processed foods, you won't reap the health benefits of a grain-free diet. Instead, choose whole foods like fresh meats, dairy, seafood, and produce. As a rule of thumb, shop around the perimeter of the supermarket, where these items are usually located, rather than in the center, which is dominated by processed foods. Better yet, shop at your local farmers' market.

    Since whole grains are a significant source of dietary fiber, some people may be concerned that they may not get enough fiber in their diet by going grain-free. Generally, if you fill the void left by giving up grains with increased consumption of fresh vegetables—especially cruciferous ones—legumes, and nuts, then fiber intake shouldn't be a problem.

    Colette Heimowitz, vice president of nutrition and education at Atkins Nutritionals, Inc., echoes similar advice to consume "lots of colorful vegetables, low-glycemic [index] fruits like berries, and nuts and seeds." Amie Valpone, editor in chief of TheHealthyApple.com, also agrees and cautions against obtaining additional servings of fruit and vegetables in the form of juice "since there is no fiber in juice."

2. **Eat mostly plants**. While the meal plan in *Lose Wheat in 4 Weeks* allows for a lot of flexibility outside of eliminating wheat, gluten, or grains, you should still strive to eat balanced meals. Because there are no restrictions, for example, on serving sizes for animal-based proteins like meat, seafood, or eggs, eating a grain-free diet may prompt people to eat more animal-based proteins than they should. Lauren Gould, a certified personal

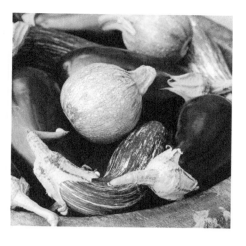

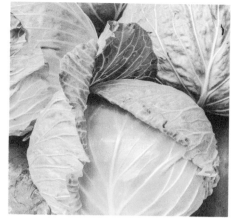

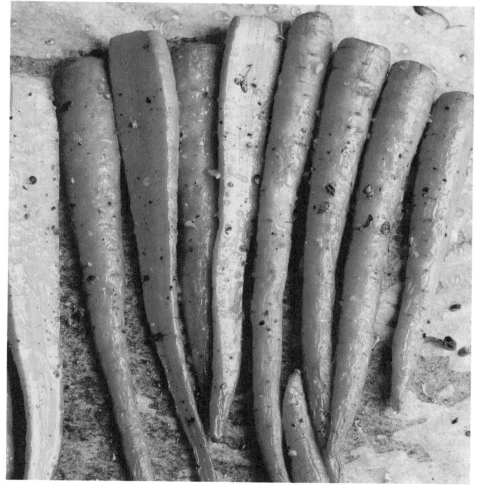

trainer based in New York and health and nutrition coach affiliated with the American Association of Drugless Practitioners, notes that some clients who go on a Paleo diet tend to consume far too much meat and too few vegetables. This can have serious implications for blood chemistry and bone health: Meat contains a great deal of acid, and without eating sufficient vegetables (which neutralize the acid), there's a greater risk of osteoporosis later in life.

3. **Increase intake of healthy fats.** Sources of healthy monounsaturated fat and omega-3 polyunsaturated fat like olive oil, nuts, fatty fish like salmon, and avocados can help you feel satiated throughout the day, reducing the between-meal cravings for snacks. Eliminate or at least reduce intake of unhealthy omega-6 polyunsaturated fat. For example, most vegetable oils, including corn, peanut, safflower, sesame, and sunflower oils, are heavy in omega-6 and devoid of omega-3. According to Dr. Perlmutter, most Americans consume far too much omega-6, leading to chronic inflammation and its related diseases.

4. **Reduce carbohydrate intake.** In addition to partially or completely eliminating grain, grain-free diets also call for reduced carbohydrate intake, either directly (as outlined in the Paleo or Keto diet guidelines) or indirectly by calling for limited intake of sweet fruit and starchy vegetables (as in the *Wheat Belly* diet guidelines). This helps keep blood sugar more stable throughout the day and additional body fat from forming.

5. **It's all about liberation, not limitation.** Many people look at a grain-free diet and can't help but think of all the things that they'll miss: fresh pasta, pizza, doughnuts, croissants, and the like. To promote a more positive mind-set, think of the grain-free diet as an opportunity to get out of your comfort zone and try new ingredients, dishes, and cuisines. Some of your favorite comfort foods can be turned into delicious grain-free versions, and many cuisines from around the world feature dishes that are already authentically grain-free—no modification necessary.

Keep these five principles in mind as you embark on your new grain-free lifestyle, and you will reap the benefits: weight loss, better blood sugar control, reduced abdominal fat, and reduced risk of diabetes, heart disease, and other chronic health problems, as well as a better sense of overall well-being. All of the 150 recipes in *Lose Wheat in 4 Weeks* are true to these principles and will help you achieve your goals. In the recipes that follow, you'll find only whole foods and healthy fats like olive oil, and you will learn new ways to cook vegetables and leafy greens that will keep you excited about your grain-free lifestyle.

CHAPTER 2

Breaking Free from Grains

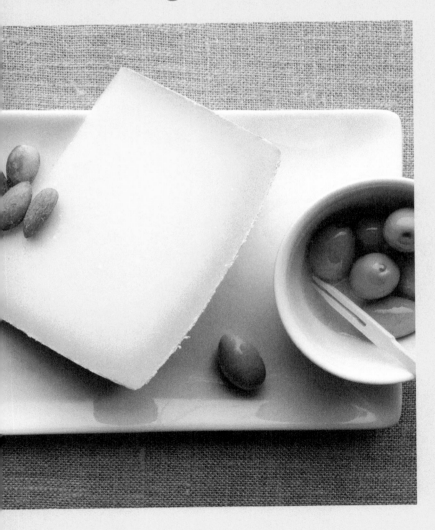

G oing on any new diet or weight-loss program can be challenging. A grain-free diet, in particular, is even more challenging because grains are everywhere—they're advertised on television, found on restaurant menus, included in many processed products, and served at social gatherings.

Five Reasons It's So Hard to Quit Grains

1. **Grains are everywhere.** "We are surrounded by ads and eating-out occasions that are filled with sweet high-carb options," says Heimowitz. And even when you're not watching TV or out to dinner with friends or family at a restaurant, just walking down the street and smelling freshly baked bread or seeing cupcakes in a bakery window can trigger yearnings for grain-based foods.

2. **Going grain-free takes commitment.** "Remodeling your eating habits—like making any major life change—takes commitment," says Heimowitz. Staying on track requires a plan that's realistic and achievable. The support of friends and family is often crucial; without a good support network, it can be much harder to decline that piece of your sister's birthday cake or to resist the cookies your co-worker brought to the office.

3. **Health claims can make shopping confusing.** "Multigrain." "Gluten-Free." "All Natural." "Fat Free." "Fortified." Walk into any supermarket, and you'll see hundreds of processed grain products touting these labels to appeal to the health-conscious consumer. Add attractive packaging and affordable prices, and you end up with millions of shoppers purchasing fortified breakfast cereals that are packed with sugar and low-fat pretzels that are packed with sodium.

4. **Cultural challenges make it hard to forego grains.** "Rice is a staple for Asian or Latin cuisines, pasta a staple for Italian," says Heimowitz. Grain-based foods and drinks are often front and center at beloved social events like birthday parties, weekend barbecues, and holiday gatherings. In such situations, eating grain-free may feel a little isolating. Plus, it can be hard to say no when you're visiting your grandmother and she offers you some of her famous lasagna.

5. **Giving up wheat results in wheat withdrawal.** "We have been indoctrinated to believe that a low-fat diet is the only healthy choice," says Heimowitz. "When you restrict fat, you get accustomed to filling up on high-carb foods like bread and pasta." Most of these high-carb foods contain wheat. As a result, millions of people have become so accustomed to eating wheat products that they actually go into withdrawal when starting a grain-free diet.

Wheat Withdrawal

When you start the *Lose Wheat in 4 Weeks* detox plan, the hardest thing to deal with may be the wheat withdrawal, since wheat most likely makes up the majority of your grain consumption. Among all grains, wheat is unique in that it has opiate-like properties and contains a compound called exorphins, which can be just as habit-forming as the nicotine in tobacco. So for the 30 percent or so of people who experience wheat withdrawal, the symptoms are very real.

What are the symptoms of wheat withdrawal, and how long do they last?
For people who experience a mild form of wheat withdrawal, symptoms include fatigue, mental fogginess, irritability, and dysphoria (feeling unwell). You may find it difficult to motivate yourself to go to the gym, take a walk, or play your favorite sport. These symptoms can start within a few hours of not eating a wheat product, and they may last up to a week. To make the transition easier, you may want to give up wheat gradually over the course of a week rather than going cold turkey.

For people with strong addictions to wheat, however, the symptoms of wheat withdrawal can be more severe, including nausea, depression, shakiness, headaches and intense cravings. These cravings may recur every couple of hours because of fluctuations in your glucose and insulin levels. Going grain-free gradually may not be an option, since even small amounts of wheat may trigger the addictive effects that you're trying to fight. The symptoms of wheat withdrawal for people with strong addictions may persist for longer than a week, though it's unlikely that they last much longer than that.

Why does wheat withdrawal happen?

There are two main reasons. One is that your body is probably used to having a steady stream of easily metabolized sugars at all times from a grain-based diet. Going cold turkey suddenly forces it to run in reverse: Instead of turning excess blood sugar into fat, it's forced to use fat stores and convert them to sugar for cells to burn, something that takes a few days to get going. The second reason for wheat withdrawal is that the brain is no longer receiving its supply of addictive exorphins.

In a study conducted at the National Institutes of Health, Dr. Christine Zioudrou and her team isolated a part of gluten that was able to pass through the blood-brain barrier in mice. She gave it the name "exorphin" in a play on the term "endorphin," the compound that's the source of "runner's high." According to the study, once exorphins enter the brain, they bind to the brain's morphine receptors, giving a similar high and creating a cycle of addiction that's difficult to break.

Using the 28-Day Detox Plan to Your Advantage

The 28-day *Lose Wheat in 4 Weeks* detox plan is spelled out in detail to help you overcome the symptoms of wheat withdrawal and stay on track with a grain-free diet. The plan has everything you need to experience the benefits of your new diet, with clearly defined goals for each week and a daily meal plan complete with recipes and shopping lists. All you will have to do is take the lists with you at the beginning of each week, complete the shopping, and follow the recipes as the week progresses.

Not only will you start to feel more energetic and focused in four weeks, but you'll also discover some new ingredients, cooking techniques, and dishes along the way.

Here is what you can look forward to when embarking on the 28-day detox plan:

Week 1: Ease into the detox. Meals for the first week contain recipes that make the transition to a grain-free diet as painless as possible. You'll start with familiar favorites that require just 5 to 10 minutes of active time and less than 30 minutes of total time in the kitchen. Recipes from week 1 include Greek Yogurt Potato Salad with Fresh Herbs (page 98) and Marinated Barbecued Shrimp (page 168).

Week 2: Explore new ingredients. During the second week, you'll ease up on classic comfort foods and start cooking delicious grain-free meals that are a less carb-focused, like Grilled Chicken Satay with Homemade Peanut Sauce (page 95) and Vegetarian Chiles Rellenos with Toasted Walnuts, Raisins, and Monterey Jack (page 154). You'll also work with several new grain-free ingredients that are relatively easy to find and wallet friendly, including spices such as turmeric and vegetables like Swiss chard. Active cooking time will increase to 15 minutes, but you'll still spend less than 30 minutes in the kitchen.

Week 3: Expand your grain-free cooking skills. In the third week, you'll encounter a few new culinary techniques that you may not have tried before but are easier than you might expect, like poaching fish in the Spanish-inspired recipe for Poached Fresh Cod with Grape Tomatoes, Capers, and Olives (page 186). You'll also learn to cook with five more interesting ingredients that are relatively easy to find and affordable. The recipes for the third week may require up to 25 minutes of active time and but will not exceed 45 minutes of total time.

Week 4: Establish your grain-free lifestyle. In the final week of the plan, you'll find dishes that incorporate everything you've learned over the past few weeks. The final week is meant to solidify an overarching principle: namely, that going grain-free isn't just a diet, but a lifestyle choice.

So, you'll find a greater mix of internationally inspired dishes like Pan-Roasted Moroccan-Style Chicken (page 222) that will help broaden your palate, inspire you to get creative, and get you started in coming up with your own grain-free recipes. Active and total cooking time will remain the same as the previous week.

Of course, the 28-day detox plan is intended as a guideline, and you should feel free to flip through the chapters and explore on your own as well, especially if you consider yourself already well-versed as a cook. See a recipe that particularly speaks to you? Go ahead and sub it in. Variety, after all, is essential to dieting successfully.

ARE SUPPLEMENTS NECESSARY?

The main concerns expressed by mainstream dietitians with respect to going grain-free, aside from fiber intake, are a lack of B vitamins, thiamine, and folic acid. Wheat products, which form the majority of American grain consumption, are fortified with these dietary necessities. But as long as grains are replaced with whole foods like lean meats, fresh produce, and raw nuts, there's no need to worry about being deficient in any of these nutrients. For example, a quarter cup of spinach or four asparagus spears matches the quantity of folic acid found in a serving of most breakfast cereals.

Seven Tips for Successfully Following a Grain-Free Diet

1. **Pick the right time to start.** "Approximately 30 percent of people who remove wheat products abruptly from their diet will experience a withdrawal effect," says Dr. Davis. Despite this, he recommends that it's best to go cold turkey because of wheat's addictive properties. To set yourself up for success, begin the detox plan in *Lose Wheat in 4 Weeks* when you know you'll be home and can prepare your own food. Don't try to start during a time when you'll be busy, like right before a big presentation at

the office or a family event. If you absolutely can't see yourself going cold turkey, you can gradually reduce your grain intake over the course of a week.

2. **Don't fall into a food rut.** "As you start losing weight on your diet and become more accustomed to a new way of eating, try experimenting with different . . . foods and recipes so that you don't get bored with your choices or tempted by forbidden treats," says Heimowitz. "Find out how to tailor your food choices based on your eating style." If, for example, you find yourself craving snacks throughout the day, you may choose to prepare something that is easy to bring with you to work, but with some slight changes to accommodate a grain-free diet. If you like hummus or guacamole, substitute your pita chips and tortilla chips with crunchy vegetables like carrots or celery sticks. Or, if you tend to get hungry just before bedtime, plan to have most of your protein for the day at dinner. Protein can help you stay satisfied for a longer period of time so you are less tempted to eat again later in the evening. The key is to keep looking for new ways to cook and new ingredients to use. Don't be afraid to experiment.

3. **Read labels.** While many of the recipes in *Lose Wheat in 4 Weeks* emphasize whole foods, sometimes it just makes practical sense to use a prepared product, especially if you need to save time. While wheat and grain products hide behind different disguises on ingredients lists—some common and confusing ones include artificial colors and flavors, caramel coloring and flavoring, Dextri-Maltose, emulsifiers, maltodextrin, modified food starch, and stabilizers—a good rule of thumb is: If it doesn't sound like food, don't buy it.

4. **Drink water.** "Thirst is often mistaken for hunger, so staying well hydrated helps you not to overeat," says Heimowitz. "Carry a water bottle with you at all times and sip from it frequently. Flavoring water by adding sliced lemons, limes, or cucumbers means you'll be more likely to drink it."

5. **Build more muscle.** "Muscle is more metabolically active than fat, which means the more muscle you have, the more calories you burn, even at rest," says Heimowitz. She advises people to start building muscle by adding some resistance training exercises into their exercise routine after the wheat withdrawal period has passed.

6. **Don't skip meals.** "Keep your hunger in check by eating three regular size meals (and your choice of two snacks) every day," says Heimowitz. "Some people do better with four or five smaller meals each day. The important thing is to keep your appetite and your cravings under control."

7. **Plan ahead.** Inevitably, you'll be invited to a party where bruschetta topped with tomatoes, pasta with homemade ragù, or fish tacos in flour tortillas are served. If you don't want to offend the host, you can try to pick out the grain products from your dish. Another possible solution is to inform the host that you cannot eat grains, or to bring a grain-free dish. Most people are willing to accommodate you rather than risk your getting sick at their party.

While the best approach to embarking on a grain-free lifestyle is to eliminate wheat and other grains entirely, some people find it easier to make changes gradually. Start by eliminating the three most common sources of gluten: wheat, rye, and barley. Then eliminate the other gluten-containing grains, like spelt and semolina. Finish the transition by removing gluten-free grains, like rice and corn, from your diet. The following lists divide the most commonly found grains and grain-like foods into three categories: those that contain gluten, those that are gluten-free, and those that are not actually grains. The last list is included so that you can make the maintenance of a grain-free lifestyle easier by substituting them for grains, since they share similar cooking uses.

Is grain-free the same as gluten-free?
No, a true grain-free diet is one that is completely free from grains, such as the Paleo diet. Gluten-free diets still allow for cereal-based grains that do not contain gluten such as amaranth, buckwheat, and millet.

What exactly is gluten?
In layman's terms, gluten is what makes pizza dough stretch, bread rise, and bagels chewy. Gluten is a protein that is found in wheat, rye, barley, triticale, and other grains.

What is celiac disease?
According to the Celiac Disease Foundation, "celiac disease is an auto-immune disorder that can occur in genetically predisposed people where the ingestion of gluten leads to damage in the small intestine. . . When people with celiac disease eat gluten . . . their body mounts an immune response that attacks the small intestine." If celiac disease is left untreated, it can lead to Type 1 diabetes, multiple sclerosis, anemia, osteoporosis, and other illnesses.

To find out if you have celiac disease, you will need to take a celiac disease panel blood test and get an endoscopic biopsy of your small intestine. To make sure the tests measure your body's reaction to gluten accurately, see your physician before you start a gluten-free diet; there must be gluten present in your system for the tests to confirm whether or not you have celiac disease.

The only treatment for celiac disease is to eat a gluten-free diet. Those with the disease must be rigorous and question the ingredients in every food they purchase and are served. It is estimated that 1 out of 133 Americans, or 1 percent of the population, suffer from celiac disease.

What kinds of alcohol can I drink on a grain-free diet?
Although you should try to limit the amount of alcohol consumed, from time to time, you'll want a drink. While beer, liquors (Scotch, bourbon, vodka, etc.), and liqueurs (amaretto, Kahlúa, etc.) are made with grains, you can safely drink wine or tequila and mescal, as long as the latter are made from 100 percent agave.

May I eat quinoa?

Quinoa is not a grain, but rather a seed. It is gluten-free and is a complete vegan source of protein, meaning it contains all nine essential amino acids the body needs to function optimally. For these reasons, this book includes recipes based on quinoa.

THE GRAIN-FREE AND GLUTEN-FREE CHEAT SHEET

While the best approach to embarking on a grain-free lifestyle is to do it cold turkey, some people may prefer to ease into it gradually. Start by eliminating sources of gluten, the protein in wheat, rye, and barley that promotes inflammation and its associated health problems. These three grains are the first ones that should be eliminated. This sheet breaks down the most commonly found grains into three categories: those that contain gluten, those that are gluten-free, and those that are not actually grains but are similar in their cooking uses and can help make the maintenance of a grain-free lifestyle easier.

Grains Containing Gluten

- Barley
- Bulgur
- Couscous
- Farro
- Kamut
- Oats (often processed in a facility together with products containing gluten)
- Rye
- Semolina
- Spelt
- Triticale
- Wheat
- Wheat berries

Gluten-Free Grains

- Amaranth
- Buckwheat
- Corn grits
- Masa harina
- Millet
- Oats (labeled gluten-free)
- Rice
- Sorghum
- Teff
- Wild rice

Grain-Free Substitutes

- Chia seeds
- Goji berries
- Ground flaxseed
- Quinoa

CHAPTER 3

Gearing Up for the Grain-Free Lifestyle

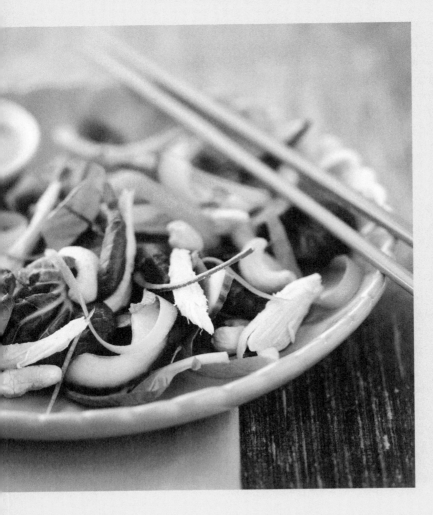

Now that you've learned the basics of a grain-free diet, let's discuss how to give your kitchen an inexpensive makeover.

Preparing Your Kitchen

Embarking on a grain-free lifestyle will likely require a few changes in the way your kitchen is set up. If you already cook on a regular basis, you won't have as much legwork to do, but there are a few things that will help you ease into the process.

The first step is to perform a full inventory of your kitchen in order to help separate the wheat from the chaff, so to speak. Get rid of (or give away) all your flour, pasta, cereal, rice, and any condiments that may contain gluten, wheat, or grain. If this isn't practical because you live with roommates or family members who are not going on a grain-free diet, then designate special areas in the pantry and the refrigerator for all of your grain-free ingredients.

When it comes to restocking your pantry and refrigerator with grain-free ingredients, Jennifer Knollenberg, nutritional analyst and recipe developer for Atkins Nutritionals, recognizes that doing so may seem like a significant expense. To save money on pantry items, Knollenberg suggests starting small. "It is helpful to purchase only a few staples to begin with, and add more as you feel it is necessary. Buy only small sizes at first. In the long run, it is more economical to throw out something small that did not work out for you." Once you've established your favorite brands and ingredients, investigate online sources to purchase bulk and specialty ingredients that may be difficult to find or cost more in supermarkets.

Essential Equipment and Utensils

If you haven't cooked much before, consider making an investment in some essential cooking equipment. It may seem like a fair chunk of change up front, but in the long run, you're not only investing in your kitchen, but also your health—and it's hard to put a price tag on that.

UTENSILS

Box grater. This handy tool makes short work of everything from zesting lemons to grating hard cheeses. Box graters are sturdy and will keep your citrus or Parmesan in a neat pile inside, instead of going all over your countertop.

Can opener. While you will be eating fewer processed foods, you'll still need one of these to open a can of vegetable broth, peeled tomatoes, or black beans.

Colander. Many of the recipes in this book call for boiling or blanching vegetables, which means that you'll need to drain them once they're done cooking, making this tool a must-have. Avoid plastic and choose stainless steel instead—that way, you can be sure it'll stand up to the heat.

AVOID CROSS-CONTAMINATION

If not everyone in your household is going grain-free, there are some steps you can take to avoid cross-contamination beyond keeping a separate space for grain-free products.

Robyn Webb, food editor of *Diabetes Forecast* magazine, says, "You should probably keep on hand two sets of equipment to separate it from any other food not being prepared grain-free." Designating a separate area of the kitchen for grain-free food prep is probably a good idea, as is keeping two different sets of cutting boards since some types can absorb contaminants. You may also want to invest in separate sets of kitchen utensils, especially when it comes to wooden spoons and bowls, colanders, strainers, and other hard-to-clean items. But purchasing big-ticket items like a stand mixer, blender, or food processor probably isn't necessary unless you have celiac disease or a gluten allergy. As a rule of thumb, if it can be sanitized or cleaned easily, most people don't need to worry.

Cutting board. Opt for one wooden cutting board for vegetables—it will be easier on your knife—and a polypropylene board for animal-based proteins. Cutting boards with rubberized feet are particularly nice since they won't slide around.

Knife block. A knife block will help protect your kitchen's most precious investment: a good set of knives. Throwing the knives into a drawer will dull their edges quickly and possibly cause more serious damage, so be sure to purchase one of these or a knife set that comes with one.

Knives. You'll want to have three knives: an 8- to 12-inch chef's knife (choose a size that you feel comfortable with), a paring knife, and a serrated knife. It's worth spending a little more on knives since you'll be using them frequently. Choose knives from reputable brands like Global, J. A. Henckels, and Wusthof.

Mandoline. While not strictly necessary for the recipes in this book, this is a nice tool to have. A mandoline is like a mounted knife blade: It can make quick work of kitchen tasks such as shredding or slicing vegetables thinly. If you decide to buy a mandoline, be sure it comes with a hand guard. Inexpensive mandolines are made from plastic and work well, but there are other professional versions made from metal.

Measuring cups and spoons. Measuring cups and spoons guarantee that your final dishes will be well balanced and tasty. Opt for stainless steel over plastic for durability. Look for sets that have a ¼-cup, ⅓-cup, ½-cup, and 1-cup measure, as well as ¼-teaspoon, ½-teaspoon, and full teaspoon and tablespoon measures.

Instant-read thermometer. An instant-read thermometer determines whether your animal-based proteins have reached a safe cooking temperature and the desired stage of doneness.

Mixing bowls. A set of stainless-steel mixing bowls is about as important as a good set of knives and cutting boards to help keep you organized after you've finished prepping your ingredients. You'll want to have at least three different sizes—small, medium, and large.

Parchment paper. Use it to line baking sheets before pouring batter on them to keep the batter from sticking. Cleanup is a snap if you use parchment paper.

Pepper grinder. There's no question about it, freshly ground black pepper is superior in aroma and flavor to the pre-ground stuff. That's why all of the recipes in this book call for freshly ground pepper. Invest in a model that will stand up to everyday use.

Sharpening steel. If you purchase your knives as part of a set, chances are they came with one of these. Otherwise, make a point of investing in one—they're not expensive, and they will help keep your knives in tiptop shape by keeping the edges aligned and ready for use. There are online videos that show you how to sharpen knives.

Slotted spoon. This is handy for just about any situation that requires separating foods from cooking liquids, a necessary step when cooking dishes like poached eggs. Purchase a stainless-steel slotted spoon rather than plastic.

Spatulas. You'll need two kinds of spatulas for the recipes in this book: a heat-resistant spatula, equally handy for cooking eggs and stirring batter, and a stainless-steel fish spatula. A fish spatula should be thin and flexible with a sturdy handle, allowing you to flip fish fillets and whole fish without having them fall apart.

Stainless-steel tongs. Long-handled stainless-steel tongs have the maximum utility, allowing you to comfortably turn steaks on a hot grill and handle larger tasks like turning a whole roast chicken. They're great for tossing salads, too.

Vegetable peeler. Since you'll be using this essential tool a lot, choose one with a comfortable grip. There are various types out there, but most beginners are generally comfortable with side peelers, which work perpendicular to the direction of motion.

Whisk. This must-have tool is used for everything from making salad dressing to Hollandaise Sauce (page 279). Stainless-steel balloon whisks are durable and easy to clean.

Wooden spoon. Sure, you could use a dinner spoon, but a wooden spoon is much more efficient and protects any nonstick pots and pans you might have. Use wooden spoons to stir soups, stews, and sauces as they cook to ensure even cooking and distribution of ingredients.

ELECTRONICS

Blender. While not essential, if you plan on making a lot of smoothies or want super-smooth puréed soups, then a blender is nice to have. When it comes to blenders, the Vitamix is king (and expensive), but KitchenAid and Hamilton Beach also make excellent models.

Food processor. Besides being great at making pesto and hummus, food processors often come with attachments that can make shredding and slicing lots of vegetables a breeze. In a pinch, food processors can be used to make smoothies as well.

Kitchen scale. The measurements for the recipes are given by volume. If you're someone who likes to bake, there's no substitute for the accuracy of a weight measurement. Choose a kitchen scale with a glass surface for easy cleanup.

Mixer. Beginning bakers will be happy with handheld models; more serious bakers will want to opt for a stand mixer. KitchenAid makes the best stand mixers.

Oven thermometer. Even new ovens can be inaccurate about maintaining a set temperature. To see what temperature your food is really cooking at, invest in an inexpensive oven thermometer for accuracy.

POTS AND PANS

Baking dish. A baking dish comes in handy for baking and roasting meats, seafood, and vegetables. If you don't plan on making a lot of sweets, ceramic actually offers better browning for savory applications and can withstand going straight from the oven to the refrigerator.

Baking sheet. Even if you don't plan on baking, these will come in handy when roasting vegetables or fish. Choose one that is thick and sturdy so that it does not buckle or warp when used at high temperatures.

Large sauté pan. This is a must-have for any kitchen. Choose a 12- to 14-inch model that is oven-safe with straight sides, a lid, and handles on both sides to help you carry the contents safely when the pan is heavy.

Large stockpot. An 8-quart stockpot or an enameled cast-iron Dutch oven is ideal for making soups and stews and for blanching large amounts of vegetables. Choose one with a lid and sturdy handles.

Medium saucepan. A 2- to 3-quart saucepan with a lid comes in handy for making small quantities of quinoa and blanched vegetables.

Small skillet. An oven-safe 8- to 9-inch skillet with a sturdy handle is perfect for frying an egg, whipping up a frittata for one, and frying a few strips of bacon. A skillet with sloping sides makes it easier for the eggs to slide out onto a plate.

Stocking Your Pantry

Once you've cleared out your pantry and refrigerator of all products that contain grains, it's time to learn what to restock. There are some surprising sources of grain in your favorite products though, so this section begins with a primer on foods and ingredients to avoid, followed by great ingredients to purchase.

FOODS TO AVOID

Blue cheese. Some types of blue cheese, such as gorgonzola and Roquefort, are inoculated with bread mold, which contains gluten.

Canned meats. If you're going grain-free, you'll be eating whole foods rather than processed ones. Avoid canned meats, such as Spam and corned beef, since they contain wheat.

Deli meats, hot dogs, and sausage. Some luncheon meats, salamis, hot dogs, and sausages can contain fillers derived from wheat.

Dried fruit. Besides having a high glycemic index, dried fruit is also often coated with flour and should be avoided.

CULINARY TIPS FOR COOKING GRAIN-FREE

The difference between a decent dish and a great dish comes down to two things: the quality of the ingredients and the techniques used to transform those ingredients. In *Lose Wheat in 4 Weeks*, you'll discover how to use both to maximize flavor and minimize shopping and cooking time.

You'll learn some important techniques that will be used repeatedly in your cooking. Since eggs are a major component of a grain-free diet, you'll learn a variety of ways to prepare them. For fish and seafood, you'll become an expert in poaching, grilling, pan roasting, and baking. You'll get a perfect crust on steaks and chops every time. You'll discover how to char vegetables on an open flame to give dips and salsas an extra dimension of flavor, and thicken soups and stews without resorting to flour. Most importantly, you'll get a sense of how to create dishes of your own. Many of the recipes in this book pair a vegetable or protein together with a basic sauce that can be modified with the addition of a few basic ingredients—spices, mustards, nuts, and fresh herbs—to transform the flavor of the dish. This level of flexibility allows you to use the recipes as more of a guideline for those nights when you just don't feel like following a recipe to the letter.

In short, by following the meal plan and recipes in *Lose Wheat in 4 Weeks*, you'll not only go grain-free with ease, but you'll also become a better cook.

Gluten-free bread. When the carb cravings kick in, you may be tempted to buy some gluten-free bread as a compromise—it may not be grain-free, but at least it's gluten-free, right? But the bread may contain rice starch, cornstarch, potato starch, and tapioca starch and should be avoided.

Jams, jellies, and preserves. Popular brands usually contain high-fructose corn syrup.

Ice cream. While it may seem that it's only dairy, some ice cream flavors like cookies 'n' cream, cookie dough, cheesecake, and chocolate malt may contain grains, so keep a watch out for those flavors. Instead try making homemade Honey-Vanilla Bean Ice Cream (page 243) topped with Strawberry Coulis (page 294) or Chocolate Sauce (page 293).

Imitation meat. Imitation bacon, imitation crabmeat, popular brands of veggie burgers (including Boca Burger, Gardenburger, and Morning-Star Farms), vegetarian chicken strips, and vegetarian hot dogs and sausage all contain wheat or gluten.

Ketchup. Store-bought ketchup often contains high-fructose corn syrup.

Malt vinegar. Although you may want to try experimenting with different types of vinegars in your cooking, avoid malt vinegar, which is made from barley.

Soy sauce. Even gluten-free soy sauce can sometimes contain traces of gluten. Replace soy sauce with Southeast Asian fish sauce instead.

Any ingredient you don't recognize. Always read your ingredient labels. Wheat and gluten come in many different guises. Avoid any products that list Dextri-Maltose, hydrolyzed vegetable protein, modified food starch, textured vegetable protein, stabilizers, emulsifiers, and leavening agents on the labels.

Great Ingredients for a Grain-Free Diet

These wonderful additions to your pantry will add tons of flavor to your meals and change the way you think about cooking.

Buttermilk. Buttermilk is the liquid left over after churning milk into butter. It is low in fat, yet has a creamy consistency and pleasantly tangy flavor that make it a versatile ingredient, great for everything from salad dressings to desserts. Refrigerated buttermilk lasts for several weeks.

Cornichons. Cornichons are tiny little pickles (gherkins) brined in a mixture of white wine vinegar, yellow mustard seeds, and spices, and they are essential to giving bursts of briny flavor to the French-inspired dishes in this book like Gribiche (page 91) and French-Style Potato Salad with Dijon Vinaigrette (page 92). You may also want to experiment with other types of pickles as well.

Feta. Brined, salty sheep or goat cheese is paramount in recipes like Greek Salad with Lemon Vinaigrette (page 85). Quality feta comes from Greece, France, and Bulgaria. It's available in blocks or already grated. Try stuffing some in chicken breasts or as a substitute for mozzarella in a Caprese salad variation.

Fish sauce. Good brands of this Southeast Asian condiment, such as Red Boat Fish Sauce, are made just from anchovies (or squid) and salt. It is a great grain-free substitute for Worcestershire sauce and can also stand in for soy sauce in certain Asian dishes. It is gaining popularity for its versatility, making an appearance in everything from Caesar salad dressing to Bloody Marys. Fish sauce can be found in the international aisle of your supermarket or Asian markets.

Fresh herbs. To add flavor to everything from scrambled eggs to potato salad to grilled meats, use fresh herbs in your cooking. While fresh flat-leaf parsley and basil are frequently used in these recipes, herbs like chives, cilantro, dill, oregano, rosemary, and tarragon also make a frequent appearance.

SHOULD YOU EAT ONLY 100 PERCENT GRASS-FED BEEF?

While eating grass-fed beef addresses a number of issues with eating beef, including animal welfare, antibiotic resistance, and environmental factors, among others, from the standpoint of a grain-free diet, it's not strictly necessary. Why? There are two main reasons. First of all, much as your body breaks down carbohydrates from any source—a Mars bar or whole-wheat bread—into glucose, it also won't be able to tell much difference between grain-fed and grass-fed beef. Meat is meat to your body; grain-fed beef isn't going to spike your blood sugar levels and cause the cascade of problems that eating wheat causes because it came from a cow fed processed grains. Second, avoiding grains from animal protein sources is going to take a lot more than just avoiding grain-fed beef. Since most meat, poultry, and yes, even fish (farmed salmon is often fed processed corn) is raised on grains, only pastured chickens and eggs, grass-fed dairy, wild-caught fish, heritage breed pork, and imported lamb would be considered grain-free.

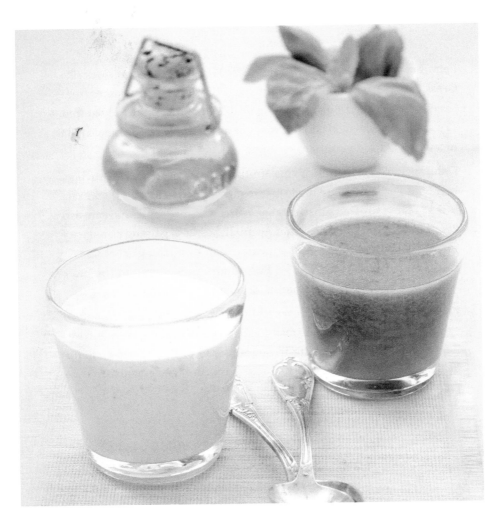

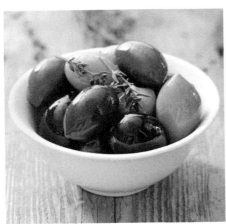

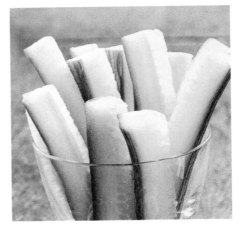

Greek yogurt. Thicker than regular yogurt, nonfat plain Greek yogurt can add creaminess as well some calcium and protein to dishes. Use it as a substitute in dishes that would usually contain a lot mayonnaise like Greek Yogurt Potato Salad with Fresh Herbs (page 98).

Olives. Olives come in a variety of colors and flavors. They are an essential part of Mediterranean-inspired dishes such as Poached Fresh Cod with Grape Tomatoes, Capers, and Olives (page 186). Many supermarkets now have olives bars where you can buy them already pitted to save time. Some varieties to try include Black Mission, Kalamata, Gaeta, picholine, and Castelvetrano.

Parmesan. Wedges of Parmigiano-Reggiano or Grana Padano are definitely worth the splurge. Depending on how long they have been aged, some have a subtle sweetness while others have a pronounced nuttiness that just can't be found in the processed stuff. Plus, you can be generous with it: 1 tablespoon grated has just 5 calories.

PANTRY

Capers. They may be tiny, but they sure do pack a lot of flavor. Capers, the fruit of the gooseberry plant, add a burst of vegetable brininess to dishes like Seared Calamari with Lemon and Capers (page 180). They come packed in vinegar or cured in salt. If purchasing salt-cured, rinse off the salt before using.

Nuts. Nuts like almonds, hazelnuts, pine nuts, and walnuts are a great way to add flavor and some crunch to salads, vegetable side dishes, and soups. They are also a great source of fiber and healthy fats. Purchase them raw and toast them yourself; toasted nuts are often dusted with flour. Once opened, nuts should be stored in the freezer to keep them from going rancid.

Olive oil. Out of all cooking oils, olive oil is unique: It is not just oil but the juice of the fruit of a tree. Because it is a good source of healthy fats, it is the only cooking oil used in this book. Purchase both extra-virgin olive oil and regular olive oil (sometimes called "light," "extra-light," or "pure"). Extra-virgin is used as finishing oil and for low- to medium-heat cooking; regular is used for high-temperature cooking.

Quinoa. Although often thought of as a grain, quinoa is actually a seed originating from a plant native to Latin America. It is gluten-free and contains all nine essential amino acids, making it a complete vegetarian source of protein. It is often served as a quick-cooking side dish, but try it for breakfast.

Tomato paste. This ingredient is a grain-free alternative to using flour as a thickener in tomato-based soups and stews like Southwestern-Style Chili with Toasted Pumpkin Seeds (page 102) and Hearty Sausage and Bean Stew (page 221). It can also help cut down on cooking time by acting as a thickening agent. Since it's unlikely that you'll use a whole can at once, opt for tomato paste in a tube instead.

Vinegar. Acidity plays an important role in balancing the overall flavor of a dish, which is why vinegar—namely, red-wine, sherry, and distilled white vinegars—play such a prominent role in the recipes in this book. Vinegar is used in everything from salad dressings to marinades.

SPICE RACK

Coriander. Ground coriander, made from the seed of the cilantro plant, has a citrusy, peppery flavor that makes it a great addition to Thai- and Indian-inspired dishes like Grilled Chicken Satay with Homemade Peanut Sauce (page 95) and South Indian–Style Fish Curry (page 191).

Cumin. The flavor of cumin is best experienced freshly ground, which is why it is recommended to purchase whole seeds and toast and grind them at home. But even ground cumin has a pronounced flavor: herbaceous and smoky at the same time. It's a major component of Mexican, Moroccan, and Indian cooking.

Turmeric. Made from an orange root resembling ginger, ground turmeric's unique flavor is suited to Southeast Asian cooking. Turmeric contains curcumin, a compound that is believed to have anti-inflammatory properties and preserve brain function in older adults.

Red pepper flakes. Essential to many Italian-inspired dishes in this book, red pepper flakes are also useful for adding a touch of heat to vegetable side dishes like Pan-Roasted Brussels Sprouts with Red Pepper Flakes and Parmesan (page 134).

Sea salt. Sea salt has more flavor than processed table or kosher salt, which is why it is the main type of salt called for in the recipes. Many sea salts do not provide iodide, however, a necessary nutrient.

Whole peppercorns. Much of the flavor of pepper is lost when it is ground, which is why you may want to consider purchasing whole peppercorns. The recipes in this book mainly use black peppercorns, but white peppercorns are also nice to have since their flavor is particularly agreeable with egg dishes and Asian cuisine.

GRAIN-FREE FLOURS

Almond flour. This grain-free flour is made from ground almonds that have been blanched to remove their skins. It's a good all-purpose substitute for wheat flour in your favorite baked goods, but pay attention to the grind: coarsely ground flours can result in soggy baked goods. You can purchase almond flour or make your own by pulverizing blanched almonds in a food processor.

Almond meal. This is similar to almond flour, but the skins have been left on intentionally prior to grinding. Its texture is similar to breadcrumbs and is good for breading proteins.

Coconut flour. High in fiber and protein, coconut flour is a healthy substitute for wheat flour in cakes, cookies, and muffins, but measuring it can be tricky. If you decide to use coconut flour, you'll probably want to use a digital kitchen scale, as it's best measured by weight and not by volume.

CHAPTER 4

Your Meal Plan in Action

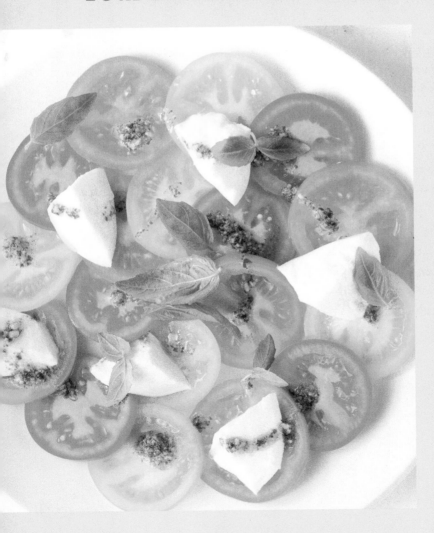

Now that you've discovered the numerous health benefits of a grain-free diet, it's time to translate that knowledge into action. Over the next four weeks, you'll make the transition from a traditional grain-based diet to one that is full of fresh vegetables, lean meats, and healthful fish.

Week 1 During the first week, you'll ease into the *Lose Wheat in 4 Weeks* detox plan with grain-free versions of comfort foods. The menu for the first week will help you stay strong in the face of cravings, with carbs still composing a fair portion of the calories, but in grain-free form. By cutting out processed foods and replacing them with whole foods, you'll start to experience the benefits of more stable blood sugar levels throughout the day. This means you'll get off the roller coaster of satiety and hunger that comes with a grain-based diet. No longer will you have cereal and milk for breakfast, only to be hungry two hours later. Instead, when the clock strikes noon, you'll only have a passing interest in lunch, and the same thing will happen at the end of the day when it's time for dinner. It's a strange new feeling, to be sure, but also a welcome one. No longer will you be living to eat; instead, you'll be eating to live.

MENU FOR WEEK 1

Day 1

BREAKFAST Frittata with Tomato and Parmesan
LUNCH Marinated Barbecued Shrimp
DINNER Smoked Salmon, Grilled Asparagus, and Quinoa Salad

Day 2

BREAKFAST Breakfast Quinoa with Honey and Cinnamon
LUNCH Pan-Roasted Pork Chops with Bean Sprouts and Peas
DINNER BLT Salad with Buttermilk Dressing

Day 3
BREAKFAST Fresh Strawberry Yogurt Smoothie
LUNCH Shrimp Scampi with Quinoa
DINNER Cherry Tomato Salad with Feta and Basil

Day 4
BREAKFAST Soft Scrambled Eggs with Goat Cheese and Chives
LUNCH Greek Yogurt Potato Salad with Fresh Herbs
DINNER Shrimp Fra Diavolo

Day 5
BREAKFAST Berry Yogurt Parfait
LUNCH Grilled Chicken Cobb Salad with Smoked Bacon
DINNER Hearty Beef Stew

Day 6
BREAKFAST Potato Pancakes
LUNCH Chicken Cacciatore
DINNER Fresh Summer Bean Salad

Day 7
BREAKFAST Italian Sausage Skillet Hash
LUNCH Greek Salad with Lemon Vinaigrette
DINNER Easy Roast Chicken with Rosemary and Garlic

SHOPPING LIST FOR WEEK 1

Canned and Bottled Items
Tomatoes, whole peeled (2 28-ounce cans)

Dairy and Eggs
Butter, unsalted (8 ounces)
Buttermilk (1 pint)
Eggs (6)
Feta, crumbled (14 ounces)
Goat cheese, fresh (1 ounce)

Greek yogurt, nonfat (3 6-ounce containers)
Milk, nonfat (1 pint)
Parmesan (4 ounces)

Dry Goods
Almonds, raw (½ ounce)
Pine nuts, raw (3 ounces)
Quinoa (14 ounces)

Meat and Seafood
Bacon, smoked, sliced (½ pound)
Beef, boneless chuck (1 pound)
Chicken breasts, boneless, skin-on (2 pounds)
Chicken thighs, bone-in (1 pound)
Chicken, whole (1)
Pork chops, boneless (1 pound)
Sausage, Italian (½ pound)
Shrimp, peeled and deveined (3 pounds)
Smoked salmon (4 ounces)

Pantry Items
Broth, beef (32 ounces)
Capers, in vinegar
Cinnamon, ground
Honey
Mustard, stone-ground (1 jar)
Oil, extra-virgin olive
Oil, pure olive
Olives, Kalamata (6 ounces)

Paprika
Pepper, cayenne
Peppercorns, black
Red pepper flakes
Sea salt
Tomato paste (1 tube)
Vinegar, apple cider

Produce
Asparagus (½ pound)
Avocado, Haas (1)
Basil (3 bunches)
Bean sprouts (8 ounces)
Beans, green (½ pound)

Beans, yellow (½ pound)
Bell pepper, any color (1)
Berries, mixed (4 ounces)
Carrots (1 bunch)
Celery (1 bunch) »

Cherry tomatoes (1½ pounds)

Chives, fresh (1 bunch)

Cucumber (1 pound)

Dill, fresh (1 bunch)

Garlic (4 heads)

Greens, mixed (4 ounces)

Lemons (10)

Lettuce, Bibb (1 head)

Lettuce, romaine (1 head)

Onions, red (5)

Oregano, fresh (1 bunch)

Parsley, flat-leaf, fresh (1 bunch)

Peas, English, shelled (4 ounces)

Peas, sugar snap (2 ounces)

Pepper, jalapeño (1)

Potatoes, baby red (2 pounds)

Potatoes, red, large (4)

Potatoes, Yukon Gold (1 pound)

Rosemary, fresh (1 bunch)

Strawberries (1 pint)

Thyme, fresh (1 bunch)

Tomatoes, beefsteak (9)

Watercress (1 bunch)

Other

White wine (1 bottle)

Week 2   You'll be adding cumin, coriander, and turmeric that are essential to the Southeast Asian–inspired dishes introduced in this week's menu. You'll also be cooking with vegetables such as lacinato kale, Swiss chard, and poblano peppers, as well as fresh seafood like tilapia and mussels. At this point, your transition period to a grain-free diet should be complete, and you should be free of any symptoms of wheat withdrawal, if you experienced any at all. You'll notice that in addition to maintaining stable blood sugar levels throughout the day and experiencing fewer hunger pangs, you're sleeping better through the night, waking up better rested, and as a result, you'll have increased mental focus and higher energy levels.

MENU FOR WEEK 2

Day 8

BREAKFAST Shakshuka

LUNCH Kale Caesar Salad

DINNER Thai Steamed Mussels with Ginger, Lemongrass, and Chiles

Day 9

BREAKFAST Blueberry, Orange, and Banana Smoothie

LUNCH Northeastern Thai Chicken Salad

DINNER Vegetarian Chiles Rellenos with Toasted Walnuts, Raisins, and Monterey Jack

Day 10

BREAKFAST French-Style Scrambled Eggs

LUNCH French-Style Potato Salad with Dijon Vinaigrette

DINNER Pan-Seared Tilapia with Olive Tapenade and Lemon Zest
Sautéed Swiss Chard with Raisins and Almonds

Day 11

BREAKFAST Berry Yogurt Parfait

LUNCH Grilled Chicken Satay with Homemade Peanut Sauce
Red Wine–Braised Red Cabbage

DINNER Quick Ratatouille and Quinoa

Day 12

BREAKFAST Breakfast Quinoa with Honey and Cinnamon

LUNCH Lemongrass Beef Lettuce Wraps

DINNER Zucchini and Yellow Squash Pasta with Hazelnuts and Lemon Vinaigrette

Day 13

BREAKFAST Eggs Norwegian

LUNCH Grilled Zucchini and Eggplant Salad with Feta and Red Onion

DINNER Baked Tilapia with Ginger and Scallions
Roasted Asparagus with Garlic and Orange Zest

Day 14

BREAKFAST Oyster Mushroom Skillet Hash

LUNCH Thai Stir-Fried Beef

DINNER Fresh Summer Bean Salad

SHOPPING LIST FOR WEEK 2

Canned and Bottled Items
Anchovies, canned fillets (2 ounces)
Clam juice (8 ounces)
Tomatoes, whole and peeled with basil (1 28-ounce can)

Dairy and Eggs
Eggs (8)
Feta, crumbled (8 ounces)
Greek yogurt, nonfat (1 6-ounce container)
Monterey Jack (4 ounces)
Parmesan (¼ pound)

Dry Goods
Almonds, raw, sliced (4 ounces)
Hazelnuts (2 ounces)
Peanuts, unsalted (16 ounces)
Pine nuts (2 ounces)
Quinoa (12 ounces)
Raisins (10 ounces)
Walnuts, raw (8 ounces)

Meat and Seafood
Chicken breasts, boneless, skin-on (1 4-ounce breast)
Chicken thighs, boneless, skinless (1 pound)
Mussels (1 pound)
Salmon, smoked (2 ounces)
Steak, sirloin (2 pounds)
Tilapia, fillets (8)

Pantry Items
Broth, vegetable (18 ounces)
Coriander, ground
Cornichons
Cumin, ground
Fish sauce
Pepper, white
Sesame oil, toasted
Turmeric, ground
Vinegar, distilled white
Vinegar, red wine

Produce

Asparagus, green (1½ bunches)
Banana (1)
Basil, fresh (1 bunch)
Beans, green (½ pound)
Beans, yellow (½ pound)
Berries, mixed (4 ounces)
Blueberries, fresh (1 pint)
Cabbage, red (2 heads)
Carrots, medium (4)
Chives, fresh (1 ounce)
Cilantro, fresh (1 bunch)
Dill, fresh (1 ounce)
Eggplant (1½ pounds)
Garlic (3 heads)
Ginger (1 piece)
Kale, lacinato (1¼ pounds)
Lemongrass (2 stalks)
Lemons (3)
Lettuce, red-leaf (1 head)
Limes (4)
Mint, fresh (1 bunch)

Mushrooms, oyster (½ pound)
Onions, red (4)
Orange, Valencia (1)
Oregano, fresh (2 ounces)
Parsley, fresh, flat-leaf
  (1½ ounces)
Peppers, green bell (2)
Peppers, poblano (4)
Peppers, red bell (5)
Peppers, serrano (4)
Potatoes, baby red (1 pound)
Potatoes, fingerling (1 pound)
Scallions (1 bunch)
Spinach (1 pound)
Swiss chard (1 bunch)
Tarragon, fresh (3 ounces)
Thyme, fresh (1 ounce)
Tomatoes, beefsteak (2)
Tomatoes, cherry (1 pint)
Squash, yellow (2)
Zucchini (2 pounds)

Other

Orange juice, freshly squeezed (16 ounces)
Red wine (1 bottle)

Week 3 This week's focus is on how to improve your culinary skills for cooking grain-free ingredients. You'll learn how to poach fish, sear duck breast, grill whole fish, steam mussels, and char vegetables over an open flame. Don't worry if you've never done any of these things before—each recipe will teach you everything you need to know for the best results.

At this point, cooking and eating grain-free should feel like second nature to you. Maybe you've lost at least 5 to 10 pounds. If so, you can expect to keep that weight off, as long as you continue to cook grain-free. Your body no longer requires a steady supply of processed sugar and carbohydrates for its daily routine, meaning you've kicked your addiction to wheat and grains. Instead, you'll find yourself enjoying healthy fats, lean protein, and fresh fruits and vegetables full of fiber, vitamins, and minerals. It's important not to lose sight of the ultimate goal—sustained weight loss—and so this week's recipes will help you stay engaged and focused by keeping your diet interesting.

MENU FOR WEEK 3

Day 15
BREAKFAST French-Style Scrambled Eggs
LUNCH Grilled Portobello Mushrooms with Charmoula
    Honey-Roasted Carrots
DINNER Poached Fresh Cod with Grape Tomatoes, Capers, and Olives
    Fluffy Mashed Cauliflower with Thyme

Day 16
BREAKFAST Berry Yogurt Parfait
LUNCH Crisp Duck Breast with Homemade Peanut Sauce
    Sautéed Spinach with Nutmeg
DINNER Steamed Mussels with Parsley, Lemon, and Shallot
    Roasted Rosemary Potatoes

Day 17

BREAKFAST Breakfast Quinoa with Honey and Cinnamon

LUNCH Kale Caesar Salad

DINNER Grilled Branzino with Easy Pico de Gallo
  Classic Succotash

Day 18

BREAKFAST Soft Scrambled Eggs with Goat Cheese and Chives

LUNCH Spicy Thai Beef Salad

DINNER Vegetarian Stuffed Cabbage

Day 19

BREAKFAST Fresh Strawberry Yogurt Smoothie

LUNCH Greek Salad with Lemon Vinaigrette
  Roasted Shrimp with Tzatziki

DINNER Creamy Corn Chowder
  Heirloom Tomato Caprese Salad

Day 20

BREAKFAST Poached Eggs with Romesco

LUNCH Cioppino
  Mexican Grilled Corn

DINNER Pan-Roasted Moroccan-Style Chicken
  Grilled Zucchini and Eggplant Salad with Feta and Red Onion

Day 21

BREAKFAST Shakshuka

LUNCH Creamy Charred Eggplant Dip
  Peach, Feta, and Mint Caprese Salad

DINNER Pan-Roasted Pork Chops with Cherry Tomatoes
  Sautéed Dandelion Greens with Garlic

SHOPPING LIST FOR WEEK 3

Canned and Bottled Items

Broth, vegetable (12 ounces)

Clam juice (16 ounces)

Tomatoes, whole peeled (3 28-ounce cans)

Red peppers, roasted (1 jar)

Dairy and Eggs

Butter, unsalted (8 ounces)

Eggs (13)

Feta, crumbled (20 ounces)

Goat cheese, fresh (1 ounce)

Greek yogurt, nonfat (3 6-ounce containers)

Milk, nonfat (1 pint)

Mozzarella, fresh (½ pound)

Queso fresco, crumbled (2 ounces)

Dry Goods

Almonds, whole (7 ounces)

Hazelnuts, raw (4 ounces)

Peanuts, unsalted (2 ounces)

Raisins (2 ounces)

Quinoa (4 ounces)

Walnuts (8 ounces)

Frozen Foods

Lima beans, frozen (10 ounces)

Meat and Seafood

Branzino, whole (2 1-pound fishes)

Chicken thighs, bone-in, skin-on (1 pound)

Cod, fillets (1 pound)

Duck breasts, boneless (2)

Mussels (3 pounds)

Pork chops, bone-in (4)

Shrimp, large, peeled and deveined (1½ pounds)

Steak, skirt (2¼ pounds)

Black bass, fillets (½ pound)

Olives, Kalamata (5 ounces)
Nutmeg, ground
Paprika, ground

Sesame seeds, white
Vinegar, sherry

Produce

Basil, fresh (2 bunches)
Berries, mixed (4 ounces)
Cabbage, green (1 head)
Carrots, baby (1 pound)
Cauliflower (1 head)
Chives, fresh (½ ounce)
Cilantro, fresh (2 bunches)
Corn (10 ears)
Cucumber (2 pounds)
Dandelion greens (1 bunch)
Eggplants, large (2 pounds)
Garlic (5 heads)
Kale, lacinato (1¼ pounds)
Lemongrass (1 stalk)
Lemons (4)
Lettuce (1 head)
Limes (4)
Mint, fresh (1 bunch)
Mushrooms, portobello (4)
Mushrooms, white (2 pounds)
Onions, red (7)

Oregano, fresh (1½ ounces)
Parsley, flat-leaf, fresh (1 bunch)
Peaches, yellow (1 pound)
Pepper, green bell (1)
Peppers, red bell (2)
Peppers, serrano (2)
Potatoes, baby red (½ pound)
Potatoes, Yukon Gold (1 pound)
Rosemary, fresh (½ ounce)
Scallions (½ bunch)
Shallot (1)
Spinach (2 bunches)
Squash, yellow (½ pound)
Strawberries (1 pint)
Thyme, fresh (½ ounce)
Tomatoes, beefsteak
  (1½ pounds)
Tomatoes, cherry (4 pints)
Tomatoes, grape (1 pint)
Tomatoes, heirloom (1 pound)
Zucchini, green (2)

Other

White wine (1 bottle)

Week 4   Now that it's the last week of your detox plan, it's time to solidify everything you've learned over the past few weeks. With practice, you'll be able to take the concepts and ideas you've discovered here and create your own dishes so that once you've completed the detox plan, you can successfully continue your grain-free lifestyle. At this point, you should feel like a new person. You've probably lost another 5 to 10 pounds at this point, bringing your total weight loss to 10 to 20 pounds in just four weeks. You've put yourself on a path to reducing your risk for a variety of chronic conditions, all of which stem from the inflammation caused by eating grains—wheat, in particular—including diabetes, heart disease, and colon cancer. At your next physical, your tests will show lower blood sugar levels, lower triglyceride levels, lower levels of small LDL (the "bad cholesterol"), and higher levels of HDL (the "good cholesterol"). In other words, you'll be just as good on the inside as you look on the outside.

MENU FOR WEEK 4

Day 22

BREAKFAST French-Style Scrambled Eggs

LUNCH Southwestern-Style Chili with Toasted Pumpkin Seeds

DINNER Pan-Roasted Trout with Pesto
   Sautéed Swiss Chard with Raisins and Almonds

Day 23

BREAKFAST Breakfast Quinoa with Honey and Cinnamon

LUNCH Garlic Hummus with Tahini
   Peach, Feta, and Mint Caprese Salad

DINNER Meatballs with Marinara Sauce
   Greek Salad with Lemon Vinaigrette

Day 24

BREAKFAST Fresh Strawberry Yogurt Smoothie

LUNCH Roasted Sweet Potato Fries with Cumin, Coriander, and Lime
   Fresh Summer Bean Salad

DINNER Gazpacho
   Pumpkin Seed–Crusted Chicken with Easy Pico de Gallo

Day 25

BREAKFAST Frittata with Tomato and Parmesan

LUNCH Minestrone alla Genovese

DINNER Seared Scallops with Lemon-Herb Vinaigrette
   Snappy Green Beans with Lemon Zest and Olive Tapenade

Day 26

BREAKFAST Berry Yogurt Parfait

LUNCH Citrus-Marinated Grilled Skirt Steak Salad

DINNER Pan-Roasted Moroccan-Style Chicken
   Roasted Beets with Yogurt

Day 27

BREAKFAST Soft Scrambled Eggs with Goat Cheese and Chives

LUNCH Steamed Mussels with Parsley, Lemon, and Shallot
   Arugula Salad with Radishes, Pomegranate Seeds, and Pine Nuts

DINNER Pork Chops alla Pizzaiola
   Pugliese-Style Broccoli Rabe

Day 28

BREAKFAST Poached Eggs with Romesco

LUNCH Gribiche

DINNER Pan-Seared Shrimp with Arugula-Walnut Pesto
   Red Wine–Braised Red Cabbage

SHOPPING LIST FOR WEEK 4

Canned and Bottled Items

Anchovy fillets, canned (2 ounces)

Cannellini beans, canned (1 15-ounce can)

Chickpeas, canned (2 15-ounce cans)

Kidney beans, canned (1 15-ounce can)

Clam juice (1 jar)

Tomatoes, whole peeled (2 28-ounce cans)

Dairy and Eggs

Butter, unsalted (8 ounces)

Eggs (2 dozen)

Feta, crumbled (¾ pound)

Goat cheese, fresh (1 ounce)

Greek yogurt, nonfat plain (3 6-ounce containers)

Milk, nonfat (1 pint)

Parmesan, grated (6 ounces)

Pecorino, grated (2 ounces)

Dry Goods

Almonds, raw, sliced (4½ ounces)

Almonds, whole (6 ounces)

Hazelnuts (4 ounces)

Pine nuts (8 ounces)

Quinoa (4 ounces)

Walnuts (8 ounces)

Meat and Seafood

Beef, ground (1 pound)

Chicken breasts, boneless, skinless (4 4-ounce breasts)

Chicken thighs, bone-in, skin-on (1 pound)

Mussels (2 pounds)

Pork chops, bone-in (4)

Pork, ground (1 pound)

Rainbow trout, fillets (4)

Scallops, dry-packed sea (1 pound)

Shrimp, peeled and deveined (1 pound)

Steak, skirt (2¼ pounds)

Pantry Items

Broth, low-sodium beef (2 quarts)

Broth, low-sodium vegetable (2½ quarts)

Olives, pitted Kalamata (12 ounces)

Pumpkin seeds, shelled (8 ounces)

Tahini (1 container)

Produce

Arugula (2½ bunches)

Basil, fresh (2 bunches)

Beans, green (2 pounds)

Beans, yellow (½ pound)

Beets, baby red (1 pound)

Berries, mixed (4 ounces)

Broccoli rabe (1 bunch)

Cabbage, red (1 head)

Chives, fresh (½ ounce)

Cilantro, fresh (2 bunches)

Cucumbers (1 pound)

Garlic (6 heads)

Lemons (7)

Limes (2)

Mint, fresh (1 bunch)

Onions, red (5)

Oregano, fresh (1 bunch)

Parsley, fresh, flat-leaf (1 bunch)

Peaches, yellow (1 pound)

Pepper, green bell (1)

Pepper, jalapeño (1)

Pepper, red bell (1)

Pomegranate (1)

Potatoes, baby red (1 pound)

Potatoes, sweet (2 pounds)

Radishes, red (1 bunch)

Shallot (1)

Strawberries (1 pint)

Swiss chard (1 bunch)

Tarragon, fresh (1 ounce)

Tomatoes, beefsteak
(3¼ pounds)

Tomatoes, cherry (4 pints)

Zucchini (½ pound)

Other

White wine (1 bottle)

Red wine (1 bottle)

Breakfast and Brunch

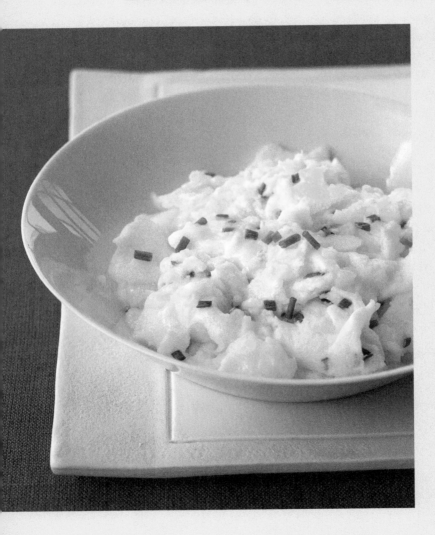

BLUEBERRY, ORANGE, AND BANANA SMOOTHIE

Nut-Free | Paleo-Friendly | Vegan

PREP TIME: 5 MINUTES

SERVES 1   *Start your morning off with this quick and easy smoothie. You'll get a healthy dose of antioxidants from the blueberries, lots of vitamin C from freshly squeezed orange juice, and plenty of fiber from the banana. If fresh blueberries aren't in season, use frozen instead. If you like a sweeter smoothie, add a tablespoon of honey.*

Diet Variation: To cut down on the amount of carbohydrates in this recipe, substitute 2 tablespoons dry chia seeds for the bananas. Soak the seeds in ½ cup water overnight before using. The seeds and liquid will form a gel consistency; add both to the blender.

- 1 cup fresh or frozen blueberries
- 2 cups freshly squeezed orange juice
- 1 banana

Put the blueberries, orange juice, and banana in a blender, and blend until smooth.

PER SERVING   CALORIES: 412   FAT: 2 G   TOTAL CARBOHYDRATES: 100 G
DIETARY FIBER: 8 G   SUGARS: 70 G   PROTEIN: 6 G

FRESH STRAWBERRY
YOGURT SMOOTHIE

Nut-Free | Vegetarian

PREP TIME: 5 MINUTES

SERVES 1   *Begin your day with this healthy, delicious smoothie, and you'll feel energized throughout the morning. Strawberries are a great choice on a grain-free diet because they are a good source of fiber and aren't too sugary, keeping the carb count low.*

- 1 pint fresh or frozen strawberries
- 1 (6-ounce) container nonfat Greek yogurt
- ½ cup nonfat milk
- 1 tablespoon honey

Put the strawberries, yogurt, milk, and honey in a blender, and blend until smooth.

PER SERVING   CALORIES: 320   FAT: 1 G   TOTAL CARBOHYDRATES: 58 G
DIETARY FIBER: 7 G   SUGARS: 48 G   PROTEIN: 24 G

BERRY YOGURT PARFAIT

Nut-Free | Vegetarian

PREP TIME: 1 MINUTE

SERVES 1   *With just three ingredients, this parfait means you no longer have an excuse to skip breakfast. For a bit more protein and crunch, add a layer of toasted chopped almonds, or for small bursts of sweetness, add a few raisins.*

- 1 (6-ounce) container nonfat Greek yogurt
- 1 tablespoon honey
- ½ cup mixed fresh or frozen berries

In a small bowl or a tall glass, alternate layers of yogurt, honey, and berries.

PER SERVING   CALORIES: 201   FAT: 0 G   TOTAL CARBOHYDRATES: 33 G
DIETARY FIBER: 3 G   SUGARS: 29 G   PROTEIN: 18 G

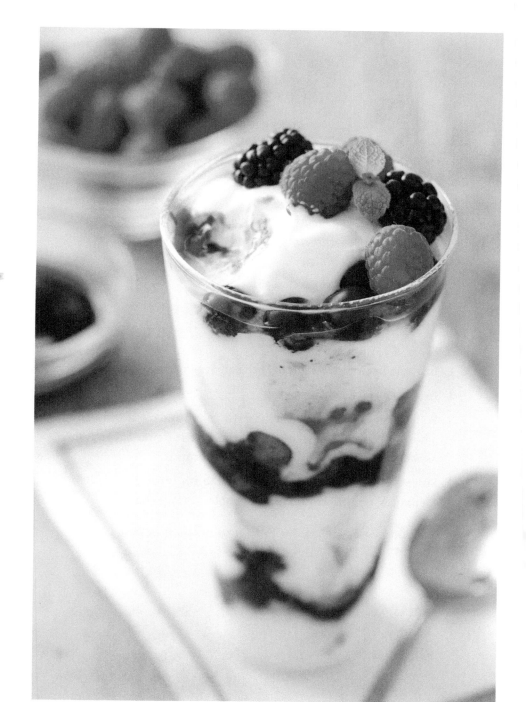

FRENCH-STYLE
SCRAMBLED EGGS

Nut-Free | Paleo-Friendly

PREP TIME: 1 MINUTE ▲ COOK TIME: 5 MINUTES

SERVES 1 *Slowly scrambling eggs over a low fire and stirring constantly makes them creamy and slightly runny. Whip up a batch of these scrambled eggs on a leisurely Sunday morning for a special treat. If doubling or tripling the recipe, use a larger skillet.*

2 tablespoons extra-virgin olive oil

3 eggs

Sea salt

Freshly ground white pepper

1. In a small nonstick skillet, heat the oil over low heat.

2. In a small bowl, whisk the eggs.

3. Pour the eggs into the skillet, and stir gently and constantly using a heatproof spatula, making sure to stir in the center of the pan as well as the edges. Curds will begin to form.

4. Season with salt and pepper. Continue to stir constantly for 3 to 5 minutes, or until the texture resembles cottage cheese.

PER SERVING CALORIES: 429 FAT: 41 G TOTAL CARBOHYDRATES: 1 G
DIETARY FIBER: 0 G SUGARS: 1 G PROTEIN: 17 G

SOFT SCRAMBLED EGGS WITH GOAT CHEESE AND CHIVES

Nut-Free

PREP TIME: 5 MINUTES ▲ COOK TIME: 5 MINUTES

SERVES 1   *There are decent scrambled eggs, there are good scrambled eggs, and then there are truly great scrambled eggs. These scrambled eggs fall into the last category, and with good reason: They are so fluffy and moist that they will practically melt in your mouth. Goat cheese and chives are a natural pairing that complements the flavor of the eggs. If you're having guests over for brunch, double the recipe and make two batches. Serve with glasses of chilled Prosecco and some roasted potatoes.*

- ½ tablespoon unsalted butter
- 2 eggs
- 1 tablespoon finely chopped fresh chives
- Sea salt
- Freshly ground white pepper
- 2 tablespoons fresh goat cheese, at room temperature

1. In a small nonstick skillet, melt the butter over low heat.

2. In a small bowl, lightly beat the eggs with a fork, and mix in the chives.

3. Pour the eggs into the skillet, and cook undisturbed for about 45 to 60 seconds, or until the edges are just set.

4. Season with salt and pepper, and lift the cooked edges upward using a heatproof spatula, while tilting the pan to allow the uncooked center to dribble outward. Do this in all directions, then scramble the eggs, and immediately remove from the heat. The eggs should still be a bit runny. Fold in the goat cheese before serving.

PER SERVING   CALORIES: 304   FAT: 25 G   TOTAL CARBOHYDRATES: 1 G
DIETARY FIBER: 0 G   SUGARS: 1 G   PROTEIN: 20 G

SMOKED SALMON, GRILLED ASPARAGUS, AND QUINOA SALAD

Dairy-Free | Nut-Free

SERVES 2   *Smoked salmon and asparagus are often paired together. Grilling asparagus brings out its slightly nutty flavor. When choosing asparagus for this recipe, select bunches with thinner stalks, which will help reduce cooking time.*

Timesaving Tip: When trimming asparagus, it's important to remove the entire woody end, but doing that one by one takes time. Use one stalk as a litmus test: Gently grasp both ends of the stalk, and bend until it snaps. That's the point where you should trim the rest of the bunch in one go using a knife.

½ cup water

¼ cup quinoa

½ pound asparagus, stemmed

1 tablespoon extra-virgin olive oil

Sea salt

Freshly ground black pepper

2 tablespoons Lemon Vinaigrette (page 286)

¼ pound smoked salmon

1. Prepare a gas or charcoal grill for medium-heat cooking, or heat a grill pan over medium heat.

2. In a small pot, bring the water to a boil.

3. Add the quinoa, reduce the heat to a simmer, cover, and cook for about 12 minutes, or until all of the water is absorbed and the hard white center of each seed is no longer visible.

4. Coat the asparagus with the oil, season with salt and pepper, and grill for about 5 minutes, or until tender and charred in spots. Let the asparagus cool, and chop.

5. In a large bowl, toss together the quinoa, asparagus, and Lemon Vinaigrette. Spoon onto a plate, and top with the smoked salmon.

PER SERVING   CALORIES: 305   FAT: 20 G   TOTAL CARBOHYDRATES: 18 G
DIETARY FIBER: 4 G   SUGARS: 2 G   PROTEIN: 16 G

BREAKFAST QUINOA WITH HONEY AND CINNAMON

Vegetarian | Nut-Free

PREP TIME: 5 MINUTES ▲ COOK TIME: 12 MINUTES

SERVES 1   *When sweetened slightly with honey and spiced with cinnamon, quinoa turns from a savory side into a hearty, healthy breakfast dish. Quinoa contains all nine essential amino acids, so it's a complete source of protein. If you want extra fiber, top the dish with some fresh berries.*

Diet Variation: To make nut-free variations, substitute pomegranate seeds or raisins for the toasted almonds.

½ cup water

½ cup quinoa

1 tablespoon honey

¼ teaspoon ground cinnamon

1 tablespoon chopped almonds, toasted (optional)

¼ cup Greek yogurt (optional)

1. In a small pot, bring the water to a boil.

2. Add the quinoa, reduce the heat to a simmer, cover, and cook for about 12 minutes, or until all of the water is absorbed and the hard white center of each seed is no longer visible.

3. Stir in the honey and season with the cinnamon. Top with the almonds and stir in the yogurt (if using).

PER SERVING   CALORIES: 417   FAT: 8 G   TOTAL CARBOHYDRATES: 73 G
DIETARY FIBER: 7 G   SUGARS: 21 G   PROTEIN: 15 G

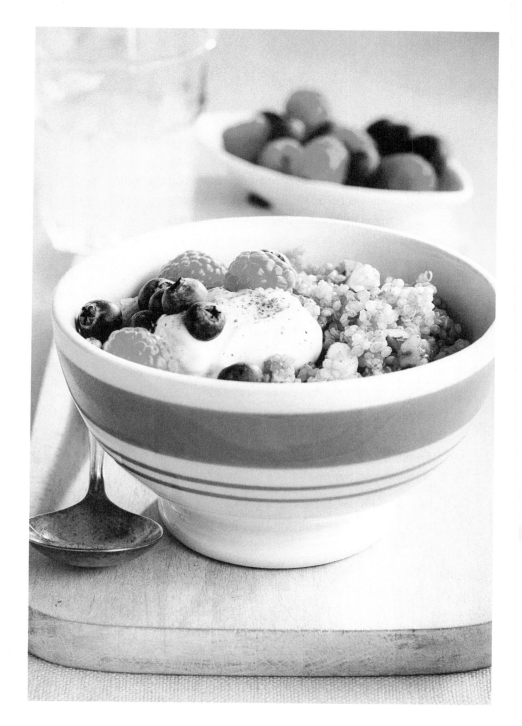

EGGS BENEDICT

Nut-Free

PREP TIME: 5 MINUTES ▲ COOK TIME: 10 MINUTES

SERVES 1   *Brunch just wouldn't be brunch without eggs Benedict—poached eggs and Canadian bacon on English muffins and topped with lemony hollandaise sauce. You'll notice that this recipe uses regular bacon to help cut down on your weekly shopping, but if you prefer Canadian bacon, go for it.*

Poaching eggs is quick and easy. The trick is to put a bit of vinegar in the poaching water to help the egg whites solidify into one piece rather than a huge mess. You'll have to leave out the English muffin, of course, but don't fret—whip up a batch of Roasted Rosemary Potatoes (page 135) to go with this dish instead.

4 cups water

1 tablespoon distilled white vinegar

2 bacon strips

2 eggs

Sea salt

Freshly ground white pepper

2 tablespoons Hollandaise Sauce (page 279)

1. In a medium pot, bring the water and the vinegar to a gentle simmer. The water is almost the right temperature when small bubbles start to form at the bottom and float to the top.

2. Meanwhile, in a medium skillet, cook the bacon over medium heat for 3 minutes, then turn and cook the other side for 2 minutes, or until both sides are crisp.

3. Break the eggs into 2 separate small bowls.

4. With the back of a long spoon in the medium pot, swirl the water rapidly in the center to form a vortex, and quickly drop 1 egg into the water. Maintain a gentle simmer for 2 to 3 minutes, or just until the white is opaque and the yolk is no longer visible. Gently remove the egg with a slotted spoon. Repeat with the other egg.

5. Transfer eggs to a plate, and season with salt and pepper. Top with the Hollandaise Sauce and bacon strips before serving.

PER SERVING CALORIES: 458 FAT: 41 G TOTAL CARBOHYDRATES: 1 G
DIETARY FIBER: 0 G SUGARS: 1 G PROTEIN: 21 G

EGGS NORWEGIAN

Nut-Free

PREP TIME: 5 MINUTES ▲ COOK TIME: 10 MINUTES

SERVES 1 *Chives, dill, and smoked salmon are a classic combination and especially good with poached eggs. Serve this with a glass of sparkling white wine and a frisée salad dressed with Lemon Vinaigrette (page 286) for a light and delicious dinner.*

4 cups water

1 tablespoon distilled white vinegar

2 eggs

Sea salt

Freshly ground white pepper

2 tablespoons Hollandaise Sauce (page 279)

2 ounces smoked salmon

1 teaspoon finely chopped fresh chives

1 teaspoon finely chopped fresh dill

1. In a medium pot, bring the water and the vinegar to a gentle simmer. The water is almost the right temperature when small bubbles start to form at the bottom and float to the top.

2. Break the eggs into 2 separate small bowls.

3. With the back of a long spoon in the medium pot, swirl the water rapidly in the center to form a vortex, and quickly drop 1 egg into the water. Maintain a gentle simmer for 2 to 3 minutes, or just until the white is opaque and the yolk is no longer visible. Gently remove the egg with a slotted spoon. Repeat with the other egg.

4. Transfer eggs to a plate, and season with salt and pepper. Top with the Hollandaise Sauce, smoked salmon, chives, and dill.

PER SERVING CALORIES: 326 FAT: 25 G TOTAL CARBOHYDRATES: 2 G
DIETARY FIBER: 0 G SUGARS: 1 G PROTEIN: 23 G

POACHED EGGS
WITH ROMESCO

Paleo-Friendly

SERVES 1   *Romesco, a Catalonian sauce, is made with tomatoes, red peppers, onions, and almonds, making it perfect for a grain-free diet. Traditionally spooned over grilled fish or chicken, romesco goes well with poached eggs. The runny yolks melt into the savory sauce. Serve the eggs with a small side of cooked quinoa.*

4 cups water

1 tablespoon distilled white vinegar

2 eggs

Sea salt

Freshly ground white pepper

¼ cup Romesco (page 271)

1 teaspoon finely chopped parsley

1. In a medium pot, bring the water and the vinegar to a gentle simmer. The water is almost the right temperature when small bubbles start to form at the bottom and float to the top.

2. Break the eggs into 2 separate small bowls.

3. With the back of a long spoon in the medium pot, swirl the water rapidly in the center to form a vortex, and quickly drop 1 egg into the water. Maintain a gentle simmer for 2 to 3 minutes, or just until the white is opaque and the yolk is no longer visible. Gently remove the egg with a slotted spoon. Repeat with the other egg.

4. Transfer eggs to a plate, and season with salt and pepper. Top with the Romesco and parsley before serving.

PER SERVING   CALORIES: 365   FAT: 33 G   TOTAL CARBOHYDRATES: 7 G
DIETARY FIBER: 2 G   SUGARS: 3 G   PROTEIN: 14 G

FRITTATA WITH TOMATO AND PARMESAN

Nut-Free

PREP TIME: 5 MINUTES ▲ COOK TIME: 18 MINUTES

SERVES 4   *The beauty of a frittata, an Italian open-faced omelet, is that you can pretty much make it as big as you want depending on how many people you want to serve. Just drop two extra eggs into the bowl for every extra person and leave the pan in the oven a little longer. The frittata is done when the edges are set and the center jiggles when you shake the pan.*

¼ cup extra-virgin olive oil

4 garlic cloves, finely chopped

1 beefsteak or other tomato, chopped

Sea salt

Freshly ground white pepper

8 eggs

½ cup grated Parmesan

1 teaspoon finely chopped basil leaves, for garnish

1. Preheat the oven to 425°F.

2. In a medium, ovenproof skillet, heat the oil over medium heat.

3. Add the garlic and tomato (reserving ½ cup for garnish), and cook for about 5 minutes, or until fragrant and soft. Season with salt and pepper.

4. Meanwhile, in a medium bowl, lightly beat the eggs. Pour the eggs into the skillet, top with the Parmesan, and transfer to the oven. Bake for 10 to 13 minutes, or until the edges are set and the center still jiggles slightly when the pan is shaken.

5. Cut the frittata into wedges, and top with the reserved ½ cup of tomato and the basil before serving.

PER SERVING   CALORIES: 281   FAT: 24 G   TOTAL CARBOHYDRATES: 3 G
DIETARY FIBER: 1 G   SUGARS: 2 G   PROTEIN: 15 G

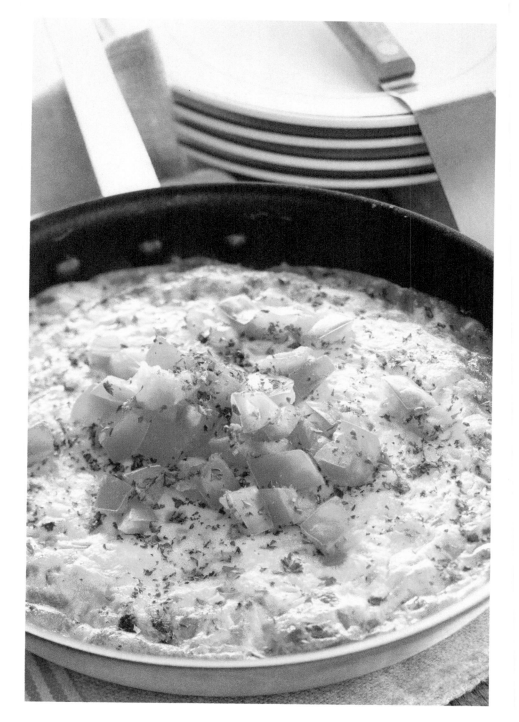

HUEVOS RANCHEROS
SIN TORTILLAS

Nut-Free

SERVES 1   *Since you're on a grain-free diet, this recipe for the Tex-Mex classic does away with the tortillas, but don't worry—you won't miss them.*

½ tablespoon unsalted butter

½ cup canned black beans, drained and rinsed

¼ cup shredded Monterey Jack

2 eggs

Sea salt

Freshly ground white pepper

½ cup Easy Pico de Gallo (page 270)

½ cup The Only Guacamole Recipe You'll Ever Need (page 110)

1. In a small skillet, melt the butter over medium-low heat.

2. Meanwhile, in a small pot, heat the beans over medium heat, and top with Monterey Jack. Stir in the cheese until melted, then set aside.

3. Crack the eggs into the skillet, and cook for 2 to 3 minutes, or until the whites are set but the yolks are still runny. Season with salt and pepper.

4. Transfer the eggs to a plate, and serve with the bean mixture, Easy Pico de Gallo, and The Only Guacamole Recipe You'll Ever Need.

PER SERVING   CALORIES: 855   FAT: 44 G   TOTAL CARBOHYDRATES: 80 G
DIETARY FIBER: 24 G   SUGARS: 7 G   PROTEIN: 42 G

ITALIAN SAUSAGE
SKILLET HASH

Nut-Free

PREP TIME: 5 MINUTES ▲ COOK TIME: 28 MINUTES

SERVES 4   *Serve this hearty hash with some runny poached eggs on top for brunch, or turn it into an easy skillet supper with a light salad such as the Greek Salad with Lemon Vinaigrette (page 85).*

Cooking Tip: Adding basil leaves at the end of cooking a dish is the best way to preserve their color and flavor.

- 1 pound baby red potatoes, cut into small chunks
- 3 tablespoons regular olive oil, divided
- 8 ounces sweet or hot Italian sausage, cut into chunks
- 1 tablespoon finely chopped garlic
- 1 tablespoon red pepper flakes
- 1 cup chopped red onion
- 1 cup chopped mixed bell peppers
- Sea salt
- Freshly ground black pepper
- 1 tablespoon finely chopped fresh basil

1. Place the potatoes in a medium pot, and cover with 1 inch of cold water. Bring to a boil over high heat, and cook for 20 to 25 minutes, or until fork tender.

2. Meanwhile, in a large skillet, heat 1 tablespoon of oil over medium-high heat. Add the sausage, and cook for 5 minutes, or until golden brown, and remove with a slotted spoon. »

3. In the same skillet, heat the remaining 2 tablespoons of olive oil over medium heat, and add the garlic and red pepper flakes. Cook for 1 to 2 minutes, or until fragrant.

4. Add the onion and bell peppers, and sauté for 10 to 15 minutes, or until softened. Add the potatoes and sausage, season with salt and pepper, and cook for 1 to 2 minutes, or just until heated through. Divide among 4 plates and top with the basil, before serving.

PER SERVING   CALORIES: 393   FAT: 27 G   TOTAL CARBOHYDRATES: 25 G
DIETARY FIBER: 3 G   SUGARS: 3 G   PROTEIN: 14 G

SHAKSHUKA

Nut-Free | Paleo-Friendly

PREP TIME: 10 MINUTES ⚠ COOK TIME: 15 MINUTES

SERVES 4   *Shakshuka is a popular dish in Israel that features eggs poached in a spicy tomato sauce with onion and peppers. This one-pan meal can be served as a brunch dish or a light dinner. Pair with a crisp sauvignon blanc or a light- to medium-bodied red such as pinot noir.*

1 tablespoon extra-virgin olive oil

2 tablespoons red pepper flakes

1 red bell pepper, stemmed, seeded, and chopped

1 green bell pepper, stemmed, seeded, and chopped

1 red onion, chopped

Sea salt

Freshly ground black pepper

3 cups Quick Marinara Sauce (page 272)

4 eggs

1. In a large skillet, heat the oil over medium heat.

2. Add the red pepper flakes, and cook for 1 to 2 minutes, or until fragrant. Add the red and green bell peppers and onion, and cook for 5 to 7 minutes, or until softened. Season with salt and pepper. Add the Quick Marinara Sauce, and bring to a gentle simmer.

3. Crack the eggs into a bowl. Slowly add the eggs to the simmering sauce and poach for 2 to 3 minutes, or just until the whites are opaque and the yolks are no longer visible.

4. Divide the vegetable mixture among 4 plates and top each with a poached egg.

PER SERVING CALORIES: 586 FAT: 36 G TOTAL CARBOHYDRATES: 49 G
DIETARY FIBER: 17 G SUGARS: 30 G PROTEIN: 22 G

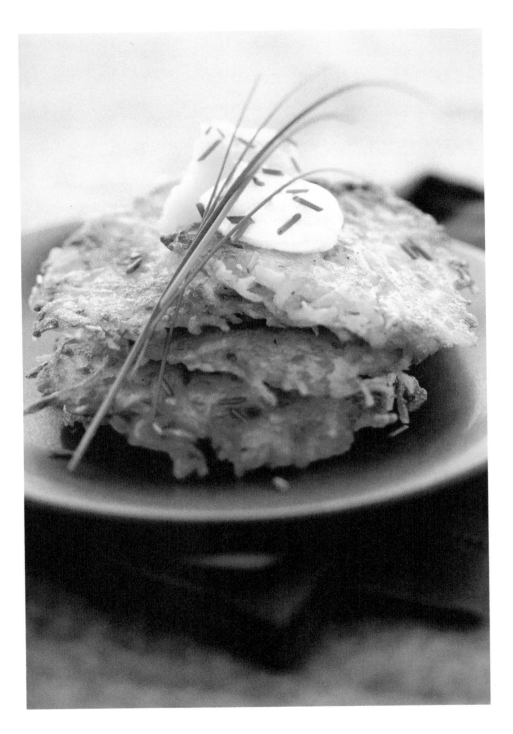

POTATO PANCAKES

Dairy-Free | Nut-Free | Vegan

PREP TIME: 5 MINUTES ▲ COOK TIME: 24 MINUTES

SERVES 4   *These crispy pancakes taste great alone or topped with sour cream and cheese. For an added twist, serve them with onion relish on the side.*

Cooking Tip: If this is your first time using a mandoline, be sure to use the hand guard, which will keep your hand well away from the blade as you work. If you don't feel comfortable using a mandoline, a box grater also works well.

4 large red potatoes, peeled
4 tablespoons regular olive oil, divided
Sea salt
Freshly ground black pepper
5 whole chives, plus 2 teaspoons chopped, for garnish

1. Using a mandoline, shred the potatoes.

2. In a small skillet, heat 1 tablespoon of oil.

3. Evenly place one-fourth of the shredded potatoes in the pan, and cook for about 3 minutes, or until golden brown on one side. Place a lid or heatproof plate on top of the pan, and in one smooth motion, invert the pan. Then, slide the pancake back into the pan to cook the other side for about 3 minutes, or until golden brown.

4. Repeat for the remaining 3 pancakes, and serve with the chopped chives sprinkled on top and the whole chives on the side. »

POTATO PANCAKES *continued*

2 tablespoons extra-virgin olive oil

1 red onion, thinly sliced

Sea salt

Freshly ground black pepper

4 tablespoons apple cider vinegar

1. In a small skillet, heat the oil over medium-low heat.

2. Add the onion, season with salt and pepper, and cook, stirring occasionally, for 15 to 20 minutes, or until tender.

3. Remove from the heat, and stir in the vinegar.

PER SERVING CALORIES: 366 FAT: 13 G TOTAL CARBOHYDRATES: 59 G
DIETARY FIBER: 6 G SUGARS: 4 G PROTEIN: 7 G

BROCCOLI-CHEDDAR
BREAKFAST CASSEROLE

Nut-Free

PREP TIME: 5 MINUTES ▲ COOK TIME: 25 MINUTES

SERVES 4   *Here's an easy recipe for the whole family for weekend brunch or lunch. This versatile casserole can be made the night before, refrigerated, and then reheated the next morning. Pack a slice along with a green salad (dressing on the side) to take to work for lunch.*

Diet Variation: To make this dish dairy-free, use a soy-based Cheddar substitute. Make sure it is free from xanthan gum, a common additive usually derived from grain-based sources, often corn. Follow Your Heart is a good brand to try.

8 eggs, beaten

4 cups broccoli florets, chopped

½ pound Cheddar cheese, shredded

1 tablespoon regular olive oil

1. Preheat the oven to 425°F.

2. In a large bowl, mix the eggs, broccoli, and Cheddar.

3. Coat a 3-quart baking dish with the oil, and add the egg mixture.

4. Bake for 25 to 30 minutes, or until set.

5. Cut evenly into 4 squares, and transfer to plates.

PER SERVING   CALORIES: 414   FAT: 31 G   TOTAL CARBOHYDRATES: 7 G
DIETARY FIBER: 2 G   SUGARS: 2 G   PROTEIN: 28 G

GRILLED CHICKEN COBB SALAD WITH SMOKED BACON

Nut-Free | Paleo-Friendly

PREP TIME: 10 MINUTES (PLUS MARINATING TIME) ▲ COOK TIME: 20 MINUTES

SERVES 4   *The Cobb salad, as it was originally conceived at the now-defunct chain of Brown Derby restaurants many decades ago in Los Angeles, called for boiled chicken. This version features citrus-marinated grilled chicken to make sure that each and every bite is juicy and packed with flavor. Neatly lay each salad ingredient in rows before adding the dressing. That's the way Bob Cobb, an employee of Brown Derby who later went on to become its president, used to serve it.*

Diet Variation: To make this recipe dairy-free, omit the feta.

- 4 (4-ounce) boneless, skin-on chicken breasts
- Juice of 2 lemons
- ¼ pound smoked bacon
- Regular olive oil, for the grill
- Sea salt
- Freshly ground black pepper
- 1 head romaine lettuce, chopped
- 1 bunch watercress, stemmed
- 3 ripe tomatoes, chopped
- 4 eggs, hard-boiled and chopped
- 1 avocado, peeled, pitted, and diced
- ½ cup crumbled feta
- ¼ cup Mustard Vinaigrette (page 287)

1. Prepare a gas or charcoal grill for medium-high-heat cooking.

2. Put the chicken and lemon juice in a zipper-close bag, shake to combine, and marinate for at least 15 minutes.

3. In a medium skillet, cook the bacon over medium heat for 3 minutes, then turn and cook the other side for 2 minutes, or until both sides are crisp.

4. Brush the grill with oil, season the chicken with salt and pepper, and grill for 3 to 4 minutes per side, or until an instant-read thermometer inserted into the thickest part reads 155°F. Let the chicken cool for at least 5 minutes before slicing.

5. On a large platter, lay the lettuce, watercress, tomatoes, eggs, avocado, chicken, and feta in rows. Toss with the Mustard Vinaigrette at the table just before serving.

PER SERVING CALORIES: 713 FAT: 49 G TOTAL CARBOHYDRATES: 15 G
DIETARY FIBER: 7 G SUGARS: 6 G PROTEIN: 55 G

NORTHEASTERN THAI CHICKEN SALAD

Dairy-Free | Nut-Free

PREP TIME: 10 MINUTES ▲ COOK TIME: 15 MINUTES

SERVES 2   *The cuisine of Chiang Mai, a region in northeastern Thailand, is known for its use of fiery chiles and lime juice. One of the most iconic dishes from that region is crunchy* som tum, *or young papaya salad, which is the inspiration behind this recipe. Since young papaya can be difficult to find, a similar texture can be achieved with fresh cabbage. The flavors of cumin and coriander permeate the chicken as it marinates, turning an everyday favorite—grilled chicken salad—into something special.*

Diet Variation: To make this dish vegetarian, substitute soy sauce for the fish sauce, and 14 ounces firm tofu for the chicken. Cut the tofu into ½-inch-thick slabs, and arrange on a kitchen towel. Place another kitchen towel on top, and place a heavy pan on top to squeeze out excess moisture for about 5 minutes. Remove the weight, season as specified in the directions, and grill over medium heat for 4 to 6 minutes total, or until grill marks appear on both sides.

1 (4-ounce) boneless, skin-on chicken breast

1 tablespoon regular olive oil

1 teaspoon ground cumin

1 teaspoon ground coriander

1 teaspoon fish sauce

1 tablespoon freshly squeezed lime juice

3 tablespoons extra-virgin olive oil

1 serrano pepper, seeded, stemmed, and finely chopped

¼ cup finely chopped cilantro

2 cups shredded cabbage (about ½ pound)

½ cup shredded carrot (from about 2 medium carrots)

3 scallions, white and green parts, finely chopped

1. Prepare a gas or charcoal grill for medium-high-heat cooking, or preheat a grill pan over medium-high heat.

2. Coat the chicken with the olive oil, and season with the cumin and coriander. Grill the chicken for 3 to 4 minutes per side, or until an instant-read thermometer inserted into the thickest part reads 155°F. Let the chicken cool for at least 5 minutes before slicing into ¼-inch-thick strips.

3. In a large mixing bowl, whisk together the fish sauce, lime juice, and extra-virgin olive oil until combined. Add the serrano pepper, cilantro, cabbage, carrot, scallions, and chicken, and toss to combine before serving.

PER SERVING   CALORIES: 426   FAT: 34 G   TOTAL CARBOHYDRATES: 11 G
DIETARY FIBER: 4 G   SUGARS: 5 G   PROTEIN: 23 G

BLT SALAD WITH BUTTERMILK DRESSING

Nut-Free

PREP TIME: 5 MINUTES ▲ COOK TIME: 5 MINUTES

SERVES 2   *Going on a grain-free diet means giving up certain things—like BLT sandwiches. But you can still have BLTs in salad form. Tangy buttermilk dressing is the perfect match for smoky bacon and hearty beefsteak tomatoes. Buttery Bibb lettuce works best for this recipe, but if you can't find it, feel free to use romaine instead.*

Timesaving Tip: A serrated knife (the kind with teeth) makes quick work of slicing or dicing tomatoes. The teeth cut easily through the skins, which prevents bruising the flesh.

¼ **pound smoked bacon**

1 **head Bibb lettuce, chopped**

1 **ripe beefsteak tomato, diced**

¼ **cup Buttermilk Dressing (page 289)**

1. In a medium skillet, cook the bacon over medium heat for 3 minutes, then turn and cook the other side for 2 minutes, or until both sides are crisp.

2. Once cool, crumble the bacon into a mixing bowl, and toss with the lettuce, tomato, and Buttermilk Dressing before serving.

PER SERVING   CALORIES: 501   FAT: 43 G   TOTAL CARBOHYDRATES: 7 G
DIETARY FIBER: 2 G   SUGARS: 5 G   PROTEIN: 23 G

OYSTER MUSHROOM SKILLET HASH

Dairy-Free | Nut-Free | Vegan

PREP TIME: 5 MINUTES ▲ COOK TIME: 30 MINUTES

SERVES 4   *With the rich, earthy flavor from oyster mushrooms and the sweetness of sautéed peppers, this dish has plenty to like. Feel free to experiment with different types of mushrooms to find your favorites.*

1 pound baby red potatoes, cut into ½-inch cubes

4 tablespoons regular olive oil, divided

8 ounces oyster mushrooms

Sea salt

Freshly ground black pepper

1 cup chopped red onion

1 cup chopped mixed bell peppers

Cayenne pepper

1 tablespoon finely chopped fresh Italian parsley

1. Place the potatoes in a medium pot, and cover with 1 inch of cold water. Bring to a boil over high heat, and cook for 20 to 25 minutes, or until fork tender.

2. Meanwhile, in a large skillet, heat 2 tablespoons of the oil over high heat. Add the mushrooms, and cook for about 15 minutes, or until golden brown. Season the mushrooms with salt and pepper, and remove with a slotted spoon.

3. Heat the remaining 2 tablespoons of oil over medium-high heat, and add the onion and bell peppers. Sauté, stirring occasionally, for 10 to 15 minutes, or until softened.

4. Add the potatoes and mushrooms, season with salt and cayenne pepper, and cook for 1 to 2 minutes, or just until heated through. Divide among 4 plates and top with the parsley before serving.

PER SERVING   CALORIES: 415   FAT: 13 G   TOTAL CARBOHYDRATES: 56 G
DIETARY FIBER: 9 G   SUGARS: 3 G   PROTEIN: 19 G

CHAPTER 6

Starters and Lunch

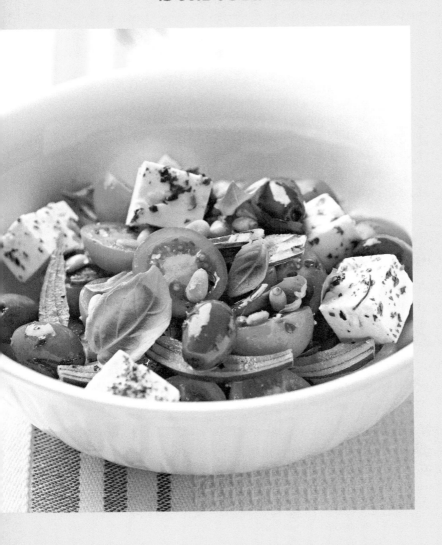

CHICKEN SALAD WITH GARLIC AÏOLI

Nut-Free | Paleo-Friendly

PREP TIME: 5 MINUTES

SERVES 4   *Traditional creamy chicken salad with crunchy bits of celery gets a garlicky kick in this dish. This salad is also a great way to make use of leftover roast chicken from the night before. If you're accustomed to adding a bit of Worcestershire sauce, which is not grain-free, try adding some fish sauce instead—it may sound unusual, but it hits all the right notes.*

Timesaving Tip: The Garlic Aïoli can be made in advance and stored in the refrigerator for up to 1 week.

- 4 cups shredded leftover **Easy Roast Chicken with Rosemary and Garlic (page 228)**
- ½ cup **Garlic Aïoli (page 281)**
- 1 celery stalk, sliced
- ¼ teaspoon fish sauce (optional)
- Freshly ground black pepper
- Chopped vegetables, such as carrots, celery, tomatoes, and cucumbers, for serving

1. In a medium bowl, combine the Easy Roast Chicken with Rosemary and Garlic, Garlic Aïoli, celery, and fish sauce (if using).

2. Season with pepper, and transfer to a small serving dish.

3. Serve with chopped vegetables.

PER SERVING   CALORIES: 709   FAT: 61 G   TOTAL CARBOHYDRATES: 1 G
DIETARY FIBER: 0 G   SUGARS: 0 G   PROTEIN: 41 G

GREEK SALAD WITH LEMON VINAIGRETTE

Nut-Free | Vegetarian

PREP TIME: 5 MINUTES

SERVES 4   *The omission of lettuce is not a mistake—it's intentional. Traditionally, Greek salad does not have lettuce in it, but since it has become so popular here in America, many people have chosen to add lettuce to it. Enjoy it for lunch or as a prelude to a main course of grilled fish or meat.*

- 1 pound ripe tomatoes, chopped
- 1 pound cucumbers, seeded and chopped
- 1 red onion, chopped
- 2 tablespoons chopped fresh oregano
- ½ cup pitted Kalamata olives
- 3 tablespoons Lemon Vinaigrette (page 286)
- ¼ pound feta, crumbled

1. In a large mixing bowl, toss together the tomatoes, cucumbers, onion, oregano, olives, and Lemon Vinaigrette.

2. Top with the feta just before serving.

PER SERVING CALORIES: 213 FAT: 16 G TOTAL CARBOHYDRATES: 15 G
DIETARY FIBER: 4 G SUGARS: 6 G PROTEIN: 6 G

CHERRY TOMATO SALAD
WITH FETA AND BASIL

Nut-Free | Vegetarian

PREP TIME: 5 MINUTES

SERVES 4   *One of the best things to look forward to in summer is the arrival of juicy, sweet local cherry tomatoes at farmers' markets. They are visually arresting—bright red, Sungold orange, cheery yellow, and even cool green. They're flavorful just as they are, but even when they're not in season, leave store-bought cherry tomatoes out on the counter for a couple of days, and they will turn sweeter.*

Cooking Tip: Use a serrated knife (the kind with "teeth") to make quick work of cutting cherry tomatoes without bruising them.

- **1 pound ripe mixed cherry tomatoes, halved**
- **Sea salt**
- **Freshly ground black pepper**
- **¼ cup thinly sliced red onion**
- **10 Kalamata olives**
- **1 tablespoon pine nuts**
- **2 tablespoons extra-virgin olive oil**
- **2 tablespoons torn fresh basil**
- **¼ pound feta, diced**

In a medium mixing bowl, season the cherry tomatoes with salt and pepper, and toss with the onion, olives, pine nuts, oil, basil, and feta.

PER SERVING   CALORIES: 200   FAT: 16 G   TOTAL CARBOHYDRATES: 8 G
DIETARY FIBER: 2 G   SUGARS: 2 G   PROTEIN: 6 G

KALE CAESAR SALAD

Nut-Free

PREP TIME: 10 MINUTES

SERVES 4   *Hearty kale is more than a match for Caesar dressing in this marriage of old-school flavors and trendy new ingredients. Serve with a mildly fruity white wine like an off-dry riesling to temper the bitterness of kale.*

Ingredient Tip: Lacinato kale also goes by the names dinosaur kale, Tuscan kale, *and* cavolo nero.

- 1 tablespoon freshly squeezed lemon juice
- 1 tablespoon red wine vinegar
- ¼ teaspoon fish sauce
- 1 egg
- 3 tablespoons extra-virgin olive oil
- 1 garlic clove
- 1¼ pounds lacinato kale, leaves separated from stems
- Freshly ground black pepper
- ¼ cup grated Parmesan

1. In a large mixing bowl, whisk together the lemon juice, vinegar, fish sauce, and egg. Continue to whisk while slowly streaming in the oil until the dressing is combined. Grate the garlic over the dressing using a cheese grater.

2. Crumple up the kale like paper, and tenderize well by squeezing it repeatedly with both hands.

3. Place the kale in the bowl and toss it to coat with the dressing. Season with pepper, and top with Parmesan before serving.

PER SERVING CALORIES: 198 FAT: 13 G TOTAL CARBOHYDRATES: 15 G
DIETARY FIBER: 2 G SUGARS: 0 G PROTEIN: 7 G

CREAMY CHARRED
EGGPLANT DIP

Dairy-Free | Nut-Free | Vegan | Paleo-Friendly

PREP TIME: 5 MINUTES ▲ COOK TIME: 30 MINUTES

SERVES 4   *This dip is inspired by baba ghanoush, a Middle Eastern egg-plant dip that has more recipe variations than it does spelling variations. If you've never had it before, it's usually equal parts creamy and smoky. You may never look at eggplant the same way again.*

Cooking Tip: Use several smaller eggplants rather than one large one. Much like when baking a potato, when cooking an eggplant whole, poking holes in it with a fork allows steam to escape as it cooks, preventing it from exploding in your oven. Yes, that's right—exploding.

Note: If you don't have a grill, you can also char the eggplant directly over a gas stove top. Do not rub with oil. Place the eggplant directly on the grate, turning it with a pair of tongs as it blackens to ensure even charring. You're on the right track when the eggplant starts hissing steam. When the skin turns charred and wrinkly all over, and the flesh inside turns creamy, it's done cooking.

1½ pounds eggplants

1 tablespoon regular olive oil

¼ cup extra-virgin olive oil

1 tablespoon freshly squeezed lemon juice

1 garlic clove

Sea salt

Freshly ground black pepper

Chopped fresh vegetables, such as celery, carrots, radishes,
    and cucumbers, for serving »

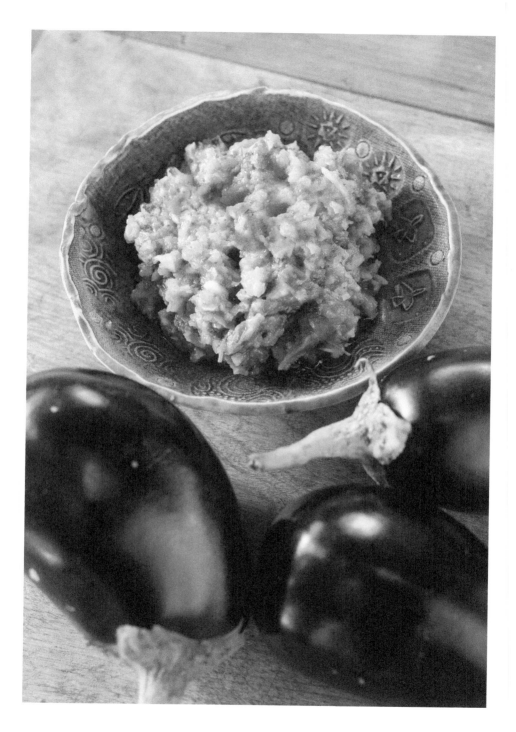

1. Prepare a gas or charcoal grill for high-heat cooking.

2. Poke holes all over the eggplants, and rub with the olive oil.

3. Char the eggplants, turning occasionally for 20 to 30 minutes, or until grill marks appear on all sides and the flesh is soft enough to be scooped out with a spoon. Remove the eggplants from the grill, and let cool. Once cool enough to handle, cut the eggplants in half, and scoop out the flesh.

4. Transfer to the bowl of a food processor, and add the extra-virgin olive oil, lemon juice, and garlic. Season with salt and pepper. Process until smooth, and serve with chopped fresh vegetables.

PER SERVING CALORIES: 182 FAT: 17 G TOTAL CARBOHYDRATES: 10 G
DIETARY FIBER: 6 G SUGARS: 4 G PROTEIN: 2 G

GRIBICHE

Paleo-Friendly

PREP TIME: 10 MINUTES

SERVES 4   *Think of gribiche as egg salad's sexy French cousin. Gribiche is often accompanied by grilled slices of baguette and flutes of Champagne. Since the baguette isn't on our menu, try Gribiche with some crudités—raw fresh vegetables like radishes and turnips.*

- 4 eggs, hard-boiled and finely chopped
- ½ cup Garlic Aïoli (page 281)
- ¼ teaspoon fish sauce
- ¼ cup thinly sliced cornichons
- 1 tablespoon capers
- 2 tablespoons finely chopped fresh tarragon

In a medium bowl, gently mix together the eggs, Garlic Aïoli, fish sauce, cornichons, capers, and tarragon.

PER SERVING   CALORIES: 286   FAT: 30 G   TOTAL CARBOHYDRATES: 1 G
DIETARY FIBER: 1 G   SUGARS: 0 G   PROTEIN: 6 G

FRENCH-STYLE POTATO SALAD WITH DIJON VINAIGRETTE

Dairy-Free | Nut-Free | Vegan

PREP TIME: 5 MINUTES ▲ COOK TIME: 20 MINUTES

SERVES 4   *Instead of potato salad with a mayonnaise dressing, a Dijon mustard–based vinaigrette lends bright, zesty flavor to delicious fingerling potatoes. Cornichons, the French name for tiny gherkins, add some crunch. Feel free to experiment with other types of potatoes besides the fingerlings.*

Cooking Tip: By starting potatoes in cold water instead of dropping them into boiling water, you'll ensure the inside of the potato finishes cooking at the same time as the outside.

1 pound fingerling potatoes

2 tablespoons Dijon mustard

2 tablespoons chopped fresh tarragon

¼ cup Lemon Vinaigrette (page 286)

Sea salt

Freshly ground black pepper

¼ cup chopped cornichons

¼ cup chopped scallions, green and white parts

1. Place the potatoes in a medium pot, and cover with 1-inch of cold water.

2. Bring to a boil over high heat, and cook for 15 to 20 minutes, or until fork tender.

3. In a large mixing bowl, whisk the mustard and tarragon into the Lemon Vinaigrette.

4. When the potatoes are done, drain using a colander, and let cool slightly. Cut the potatoes into bite-size chunks, toss in the dressing, and season with salt and pepper. Add the cornichons and scallions to the bowl, and mix well.

PER SERVING   CALORIES: 193   FAT: 11 G   TOTAL CARBOHYDRATES: 22 G
DIETARY FIBER: 3 G   SUGARS: 2 G   PROTEIN: 4 G

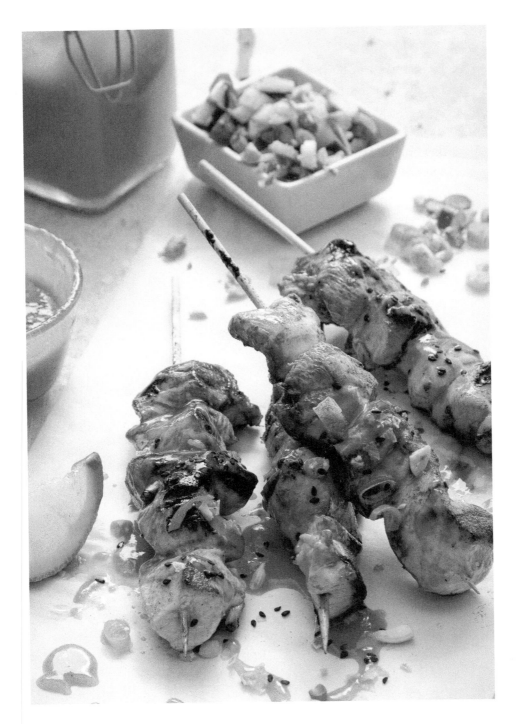

GRILLED CHICKEN SATAY WITH HOMEMADE PEANUT SAUCE

Dairy-Free

PREP TIME: 5 MINUTES ▲ COOK TIME: 10 MINUTES

SERVES 4   *The peanut sauce that comes with takeout chicken satay can sometimes be too sweet. Luckily, it's easy to re-create at home. Here, honey is used instead of sugar, and a splash of lime juice balances the overall flavor. Serve with cucumber relish on the side for an added kick.*

Diet Variation: To make this dish vegetarian, substitute 14 ounces of firm tofu for the chicken. Cut into 1-inch-thick cubes, and arrange on a kitchen towel. Place another kitchen towel on top, and place a heavy pan on top to squeeze out excess moisture for about 5 minutes. Remove the weight, coat with 1 tablespoon olive oil, season as specified in the directions, and grill over medium heat for 4 to 6 minutes total, or until grill marks appear on both sides.

Sea salt
1 teaspoon ground coriander
1 teaspoon ground turmeric
1 pound boneless, skinless chicken thighs, cut into chunks
½ cup Homemade Peanut Sauce (page 292)

1. Prepare a gas or charcoal grill for medium-high-heat cooking. If using wooden skewers, soak them in water for about 15 minutes.

2. In a small bowl, combine the salt, coriander, and turmeric. Add the chicken and toss well. Thread the chicken onto the skewers, and grill, turning once, for 3 to 4 minutes per side, or until cooked through and the internal temperature reaches 155°F on an instant-read thermometer.

3. Serve with the Homemade Peanut Sauce and cucumber relish (if using) on the side. »

FOR THE CUCUMBER RELISH (IF USING)

2 teaspoons fish sauce

1 teaspoon distilled white vinegar

1 teaspoon honey

½ cup chopped cucumber

1 tablespoon finely chopped shallot

1 red Thai chile, stemmed, seeded, and finely chopped

2 tablespoons finely chopped scallions, green and white parts

¼ teaspoon black sesame seeds

1. In a small bowl, stir together the fish sauce, vinegar, and honey until well blended.

2. Add the cucumber, shallot, chile, scallions, and sesame seeds, and toss to combine.

PER SERVING CALORIES: 337 FAT: 18 G TOTAL CARBOHYDRATES: 8 G
DIETARY FIBER: 2 G SUGARS: 5 G PROTEIN: 38 G

BABY SHRIMP CEVICHE WITH MANGO, RADISH, AND RED ONION

Nut-Free | Paleo-Friendly

PREP TIME: 10 MINUTES ▲ COOK TIME: 15 MINUTES

SERVES 4   *Ceviche is a mixture of different types of fresh seafood (fish, shrimp, and calamari) that is marinated in citrus juices and chiles and topped with red onion and cilantro. In Peru, it's usually served with a bit of steamed sweet potato and corn. This tropically inspired version of ceviche uses mango and thinly sliced radish for sweetness and crunch. Don't marinate the seafood for more than 15 minutes, or else it will toughen and become too chewy.*

Diet Variation: To make this dish vegetarian, substitute 1 pound finely diced white button mushrooms or cremini mushrooms. Steam the mushrooms for about 10 minutes, then marinate with the remaining ingredients as specified in the directions.

1 pound baby (or about 90- to 110-count per pound) shrimp,
   peeled and deveined
½ cup finely diced ripe mango
3 red radishes, thinly sliced
¼ cup thinly sliced red onion
1 tablespoon finely chopped cilantro (optional)
1 jalapeño pepper, stemmed, seeded, and finely chopped (optional)
Juice of 1 lime
Sea salt

1. In a mixing bowl, toss together the shrimp, mango, radishes, onion, cilantro (if using), jalapeño (if using), and lime juice.

2. Season with salt, and refrigerate for 15 minutes before serving.

PER SERVING   CALORIES: 113   FAT: 1 G   TOTAL CARBOHYDRATES: 8 G
DIETARY FIBER: 1 G   SUGARS: 6 G   PROTEIN: 20 G

GREEK YOGURT POTATO SALAD WITH FRESH HERBS

Nut-Free | Vegetarian

PREP TIME: 5 MINUTES ▲ COOK TIME: 25 MINUTES

SERVES 4   *If there's a backyard party involving a grill and friends and family, you can be sure that potato salad will be on the menu. But traditional potato salad, often made with an unholy amount of store-bought mayonnaise, is a dieter's nightmare. This slimmed-down version retains much of the same great flavor and creaminess while cutting out the calories and fat. Use whatever herbs you like for this salad—dill and chives are a particularly good combination.*

Ingredient Tip: Look for similar size potatoes at the store to ensure even cooking.

1 pound baby red or Yukon Gold potatoes

¼ cup extra-virgin olive oil

1 tablespoon freshly squeezed lemon juice

1 (6-ounce) container nonfat Greek yogurt

2 tablespoons chopped fresh dill

2 tablespoons chopped fresh chives

Sea salt

Freshly ground black pepper

1. Place the potatoes in a medium pot, and cover with 1 inch of cold water.

2. Bring to a boil over high heat, and cook for 20 to 25 minutes, or until fork tender.

3. In a medium bowl, slowly whisk the oil into the lemon juice until combined, then whisk in the yogurt. Add the dill and chives, and season with salt and pepper.

4. When the potatoes are done, drain using a colander, and let cool. Once cool enough to handle, cut the potatoes into bite-size chunks, and place in a bowl. Toss with the dressing and season with additional salt and pepper before serving.

PER SERVING CALORIES: 233 FAT: 13 G TOTAL CARBOHYDRATES: 27 G
DIETARY FIBER: 2 G SUGARS: 6 G PROTEIN: 6 G

ROASTED BEETS
WITH YOGURT

Nut-Free | Vegetarian

PREP TIME: 5 MINUTES ▲ COOK TIME: 40 MINUTES

SERVES 4   *A classic combination, roasted beet and yogurt salads are popular throughout the Mediterranean. Serve with some Charmoula (page 283) on the side if you want to add a zesty Moroccan flavor to the dish.*

Diet Variation: To make this dish dairy-free, use a soy-based yogurt substitute instead of the Greek yogurt. Look for brands that are free from stabilizers, thickeners, and grain-based additives such as cornstarch and rice starch. Stonyfield Organic is a good brand to try.

- 1 pound baby beets, trimmed
- 2 tablespoons regular olive oil
- Sea salt
- ¼ cup nonfat Greek yogurt

1. Preheat the oven to 475°F.

2. In a medium bowl, toss the beets with the oil, and season with salt.

3. Wrap each beet in aluminum foil, and place on a baking sheet. Roast in the oven for about 40 minutes, or until the beets can be pierced through with a fork. Remove from the oven, let cool, and unwrap.

4. Chop into bite-size chunks, place in a medium bowl, and spoon yogurt on top before serving.

PER SERVING CALORIES: 195 FAT: 16 G TOTAL CARBOHYDRATES: 11 G
DIETARY FIBER: 3 G SUGARS: 8 G PROTEIN: 4 G

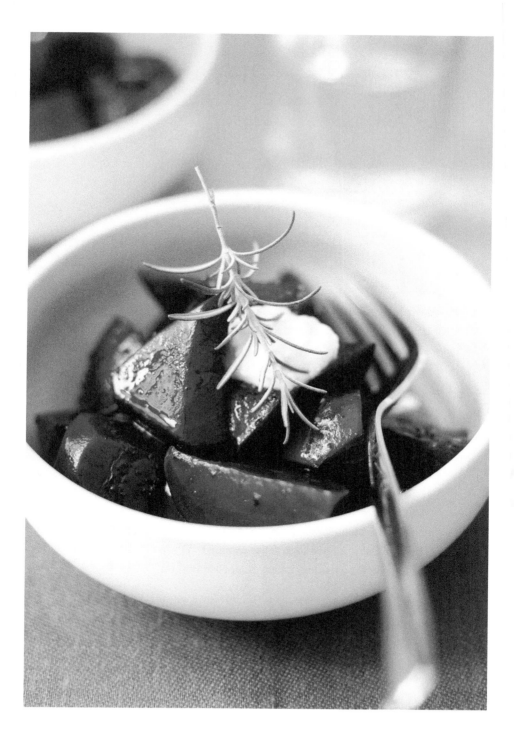

SOUTHWESTERN-STYLE CHILI WITH TOASTED PUMPKIN SEEDS

Nut-Free

PREP TIME: 7 MINUTES ▲ COOK TIME: 38 MINUTES

SERVES 4 *Although chili is often thought of as an all-day project, much of the cooking time is actually spent thickening the base. To help speed the process, this recipe calls for puréeing the beans and potatoes and adding them back to the mix.*

Diet Variation: This chili can be made vegetarian. Instead of 1 pound ground pork, substitute 1 pound mixed mushrooms and cook for 10 to 15 minutes instead, or until golden brown. Replace the beef broth with vegetable broth.

1 tablespoon regular olive oil

1 pound ground pork

Sea salt

Freshly ground black pepper

1 red onion, chopped

3 garlic cloves, chopped

1 jalapeño pepper, stemmed, seeded, and chopped

1 tablespoon tomato paste

2 quarts (8 cups) low-sodium beef broth

1 pound baby red potatoes, finely chopped

1 (15-ounce) can kidney beans, drained and rinsed

1. In a large pot, heat the oil over medium-high heat.

2. Sear the pork for 5 minutes, or until browned, breaking up large chunks, and season with salt and pepper.

3. Add the onion, garlic, and jalapeño, and cook for 2 to 3 minutes, or until fragrant. Season with salt and pepper. Add the tomato paste, and cook for 1 minute, or until fragrant. Add the broth, season with salt and pepper, and increase the heat to high. When the mixture reaches a boil, add the potatoes, and cook for 20 to 25 minutes, or until the potatoes are fork tender.

4. Place the beans and 1 cup of the chili (making sure to get as many potatoes as possible) in the bowl of a food processor, and process until blended.

5. Transfer the mixture back to the pot, and simmer for 3 to 4 minutes, or until thickened.

6. Divide among 4 bowls and serve hot.

PER SERVING CALORIES: 436 FAT: 6 G TOTAL CARBOHYDRATES: 15 G
DIETARY FIBER: 12 G SUGARS: 3 G PROTEIN: 38 G

FRESH SUMMER
BEAN SALAD

Vegetarian

PREP TIME: 10 MINUTES ▲ COOK TIME: 5 MINUTES

SERVES 4   *Snappy green and yellow fresh beans make a great pairing with ripe cherry tomatoes and pine nuts in this salad. Haricots verts are slender French green beans with smaller seeds and a more delicate flavor than regular green beans. If you can't find haricots verts or yellow beans, it's fine to use green beans instead.*

Ingredient Tip: Extend the shelf life of fresh herbs by trimming the stems, standing them in a small jar of water, covering the leaves with a loose plastic bag, and storing the jar in the refrigerator. For a simpler solution, wrap the herbs in a damp paper towel before putting them in the refrigerator.

Sea salt

½ pound haricots verts, trimmed

½ pound yellow wax beans, trimmed

½ pound ripe cherry tomatoes, halved

¼ pound feta, crumbled

¼ cup pine nuts, toasted

3 tablespoons Lemon Vinaigrette (page 286)

Freshly ground black pepper

¼ cup chopped basil

1. Bring a large pot of salted water to a boil over high heat. Fill a large mixing bowl with ice water.

2. Add the haricots verts and yellow wax beans, and cook for about 2 minutes, or until crisp-tender (they should retain their color). Drain the beans and then immediately submerge them in the ice water for 2 minutes to stop the cooking. Drain well.

3. Dry the mixing bowl, and toss together the beans, tomatoes, feta, pine nuts, and Lemon Vinaigrette. Season with pepper, and top with the basil just before serving.

PER SERVING CALORIES: 222 FAT: 19 G TOTAL CARBOHYDRATES: 10 G
DIETARY FIBER: 4 G SUGARS: 5 G PROTEIN: 7 G

LEMONGRASS BEEF LETTUCE WRAPS

Nut-Free | Paleo-Friendly

PREP TIME: 20 MINUTES ▲ COOK TIME: 15 MINUTES

SERVES 4   *These lettuce wraps are inspired by Vietnamese summer rolls, which are filled with lettuce, pickled carrot and daikon radish, rice vermicelli noodles, and thin slices of pork pâté. The wrapping is usually made out of steamed rice paper. Here, we take similar ingredients and put them into a lettuce wrap to make a grain-free version that is equally delicious.*

Cooking Tip: To make equal-size wraps, tear larger leaves into smaller pieces.

- 1 lemongrass stalk
- 3 tablespoons fish sauce, divided
- 3 tablespoons honey, divided
- Juice of 2 limes
- 1 tablespoon toasted sesame oil
- 1 pound sirloin steak
- 2 tablespoons water
- 1 head red-leaf or green-leaf lettuce, leaves removed
- 1 cup mint leaves
- 1 cup cilantro sprigs
- 1 cup shredded carrot

1. Remove and discard the tough outer layers of the lemongrass stalk, and thinly slice the tender core.

2. Place the lemongrass, 1 tablespoon of fish sauce, 1 tablespoon of honey, lime juice, sesame oil, and steak in a 1-gallon zipper-close bag; seal and shake to mix well.

3. Prepare a gas or charcoal grill for high-heat cooking. Remove the meat from the marinade after about 15 minutes, and place on the grill. Cook until the desired level of doneness is reached—for medium rare, about 3 minutes per side. Let the steak rest for at least 5 minutes before slicing.

4. In a small bowl, mix together the remaining 2 tablespoons of fish sauce, remaining 2 tablespoons of honey, and water to make the dipping sauce.

5. To make a lettuce wrap, take a lettuce leaf, place a few slices of beef, some mint leaves, cilantro sprigs, and shredded carrot on it, roll, and tuck the sides underneath.

PER SERVING CALORIES: 337 FAT: 11 G TOTAL CARBOHYDRATES: 24 G
DIETARY FIBER: 4 G SUGARS: 17 G PROTEIN: 37 G

Snacks and Sides

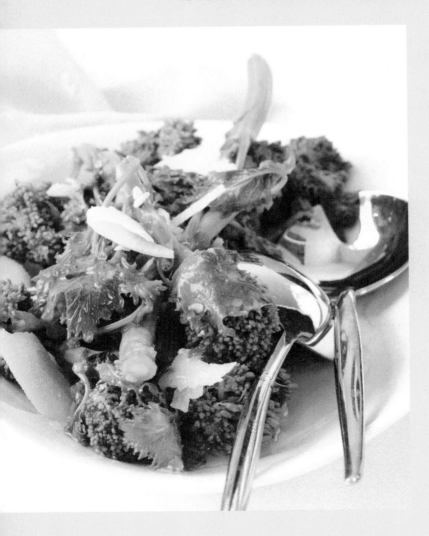

THE ONLY GUACAMOLE
RECIPE YOU'LL EVER NEED

Dairy-Free | Nut-Free | Paleo-Friendly | Vegan

PREP TIME: 5 MINUTES

SERVES 4   *Traditional guacamole should be neither chunky nor completely smooth. A good guacamole should have a balance somewhere in between. Why? In Mexico, guacamole is made with something similar to a mortar-and-pestle, called a molcajete. The important thing is that the molcajete allows the guacamole to retain some texture, mostly smooth, but with a few chunks of recognizable avocado here and there. There's no need to run out and buy one, though: Judicious use of a fork and a bowl will do almost as well. Just please don't use a food processor.*

Ingredient Tip: *Place unripe avocados in a paper bag for a day or two to ripen. They are ready to be used when they yield slightly to gentle pressure.*

2 ripe Haas avocados

Juice of 1 lime

¼ cup finely chopped cilantro

1 jalapeño pepper, stemmed, seeded, and finely diced (optional)

Sea salt

Freshly ground black pepper

1. Hold 1 avocado in one hand, and rotate it while tracing a line along the long end all the way through to the pit using a chef's knife. Twist the two halves apart. Holding the half with the pit in one hand, carefully bury the blade of the knife into the pit, and twist to remove. Using a spoon, scoop the flesh out of the halves into a medium bowl. Repeat with the other avocado.

2. Add the lime juice, cilantro, and jalapeño (if using), and mash using a fork or spoon until creamy but with small chunks remaining. Season with salt and pepper before serving.

PER SERVING   CALORIES: 211   FAT: 20 G   TOTAL CARBOHYDRATES: 11 G
DIETARY FIBER: 7 G   SUGARS: 1 G   PROTEIN: 2 G

FRESH
ARTICHOKE-LEMON DIP

Dairy-Free | Nut-Free | Paleo-Friendly | Vegan

PREP TIME: 20 MINUTES ▲ COOK TIME: 15 MINUTES

SERVES 4 *Most artichoke dip recipes make use of frozen or canned artichoke hearts, which is okay, but you're not going for just okay here. Trimming artichokes is not difficult: a sharp knife, a small spoon, and a bit of practice are all that's needed. This dip is definitely worth the effort. Serve with some chopped radishes, carrots, and celery for a healthy snack.*

Juice of 3 lemons, divided

2 globe artichokes

½ cup extra-virgin olive oil

Sea salt

Freshly ground black pepper

1. In a pot large enough to fit both artichokes, bring 2 inches of water to a boil; fill a medium bowl with water, and squeeze 2 lemons into it.

2. Using a pair of kitchen shears, take one of the artichokes, and snip off the pointy ends of the leaves. Using a serrated knife, slice off and discard the top one-third of the artichoke, and dip the rest of the artichoke in the lemon water to prevent discoloration. Using your fingers, snap off the tough outer leaves until you reach the tender, bright green ones on the inside, and cut each artichoke in half lengthwise. Place one half in the lemon water. Using a small spoon, scoop out and discard the pointy thistles in the center of the artichoke (don't be afraid to get aggressive). Place the artichoke half in the lemon water, repeat with the other half, and trim the other artichoke the same way. »

3. Place the artichokes cut side down in the boiling water, and cook, covered, for 12 to 13 minutes, or until the hearts are tender. Drain the artichokes, and when cool enough to handle, discard the outer leaves (they should just fall right off, leaving the heart).

4. Place the artichoke hearts, the remaining juice of 1 lemon, and the oil in the bowl of a food processor, and blend until smooth. Season with salt and pepper before serving.

PER SERVING   CALORIES: 258   FAT: 25 G   TOTAL CARBOHYDRATES: 10 G
DIETARY FIBER: 5 G   SUGARS: 1 G   PROTEIN: 3 G

PUGLIESE-STYLE BROCCOLI RABE

Dairy-Free | Nut-Free | Paleo-Friendly

PREP TIME: 5 MINUTES ▲ COOK TIME: 15 MINUTES

SERVES 4   *The region of Puglia is located on the heel of Italy's boot. One traditional dish is* orecchiette con cime di rapa, *or small ear-shaped pasta shells topped with broccoli rabe, anchovies, garlic, and plenty of red pepper flakes. Without the pasta, the broccoli rabe is a zesty side dish.*

Ingredient Tip: Broccoli rabe, also sold as rapini, is often confused with broccolini, which has a similar appearance. The two vegetables are unrelated and have different flavors; broccolini lacks the bitterness that makes broccoli rabe special.

Sea salt

1 bunch broccoli rabe, trimmed

2 tablespoons extra-virgin olive oil

2 anchovy fillets, finely chopped

1 tablespoon red pepper flakes

3 garlic cloves, thinly sliced

1. Bring a large pot of salted water to a boil over high heat, and fill a large bowl with ice water.

2. Add the broccoli rabe to the pot, and cook for 2 to 3 minutes, or until bright green and crisp-tender. Transfer to the ice water using tongs, drain, and pat dry. Chop into bite-size pieces.

3. In a large skillet, heat the oil over medium heat. Add the anchovy fillets, red pepper flakes, and garlic, and cook for 3 to 4 minutes, or until the garlic is golden brown. Add the broccoli rabe.

4. Cook, stirring regularly, for 5 to 7 minutes, until tender. Season with salt before serving.

PER SERVING   CALORIES: 102   FAT: 8 G   TOTAL CARBOHYDRATES: 6 G
DIETARY FIBER: 1 G   SUGARS: 0 G   PROTEIN: 4 G

GARLIC HUMMUS
WITH TAHINI

Dairy-Free | Nut-Free | Vegan

PREP TIME: 5 MINUTES

SERVES 8   *Tahini is ground toasted sesame seeds and can be easily found in most grocery stores. This one ingredient is what makes hummus unique. If you're not a fan of raw garlic, feel free to leave it out, but it rounds out the hummus nicely.*

Although hummus is typically served with pita or chips, try serving it with some chopped radishes, celery, carrots, or jicama instead for a satisfying crunch with each bite.

- **1 (15-ounce can) chickpeas, drained and rinsed**
- **1 garlic clove**
- **Juice of 1½ lemons**
- **1 cup extra-virgin olive oil**
- **½ cup tahini**
- **Sea salt**
- **Freshly ground black pepper**
- **Chopped vegetables, such as carrots, celery, tomatoes, and cucumbers, for serving**

1. In the bowl of a food processor, put the chickpeas, garlic, and lemon juice.

2. With the machine running, add the oil and tahini until the mixture becomes a smooth paste.

3. Season with salt and pepper and pulse to combine.

4. Serve with the chopped vegetables.

PER SERVING   CALORIES: 502   FAT: 37 G   TOTAL CARBOHYDRATES: 37 G
DIETARY FIBER: 11 G   SUGARS: 6 G   PROTEIN: 13 G

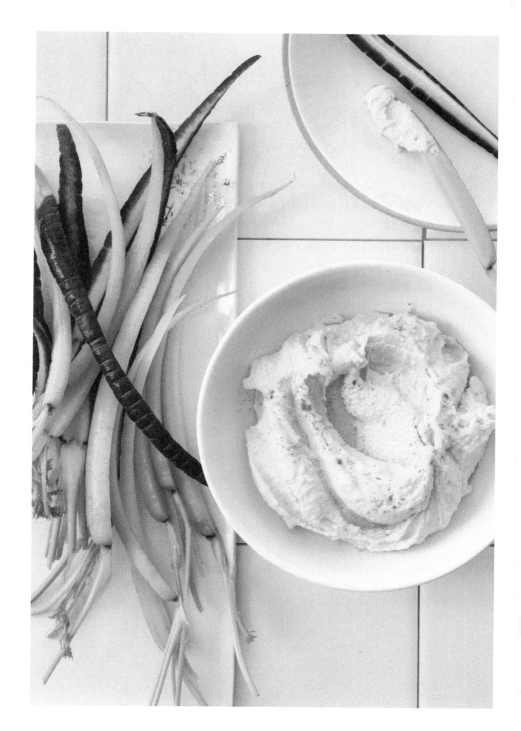

CLASSIC SUCCOTASH

Dairy-Free | Nut-Free | Paleo-Friendly | Vegan

PREP TIME: 10 MINUTES ▲ COOK TIME: 15 MINUTES

SERVES 4   *The name of this dish comes from the Narragansett Indian word msickquatash. The combination of sweet corn, earthy lima beans, bell peppers, and zucchini is one that goes well with barbecued chicken or grilled salmon.*

- **2 ears fresh corn (or about 1½ cups frozen corn, thawed)**
- **1 tablespoon extra-virgin olive oil**
- **1 cup finely diced red onion**
- **1 red bell pepper, finely diced**
- **1 zucchini, finely diced**
- **10 ounces frozen lima beans, thawed**
- **Sea salt**
- **Freshly ground black pepper**

1. Remove the kernels from the corn by placing the flat end of each ear on a firm surface and slicing down each side with a chef's knife.

2. In a large skillet, heat the oil over medium heat.

3. Add the onion, bell pepper, and zucchini and cook for 3 to 4 minutes, or until fragrant and crisp-tender.

4. Add the corn and lima beans, and cook for 5 to 7 minutes, or until fragrant and crisp-tender.

5. Season with salt and pepper before serving.

PER SERVING   CALORIES: 169   FAT: 5 G   TOTAL CARBOHYDRATES: 27 G
DIETARY FIBER: 6 G   SUGARS: 6 G   PROTEIN: 7 G

MEXICAN GRILLED CORN

Nut-Free | Vegetarian

PREP TIME: 5 MINUTES ▲ COOK TIME: 15 MINUTES

SERVES 4   Elotes callejeros, *or grilled corn, is a popular Mexican street food that has made its way north. Once grilled, each ear is slathered with queso fresco, butter, and lime. So simple, so delicious. If queso fresco or cotija is difficult to find, you can substitute feta instead, which is also delicious.*

Diet Variation: To make this dish dairy-free, use a soy-based Monterey Jack or mozzarella instead of the queso fresco or cotija cheese called for in the recipe. Make sure it is free from xanthan gum, a common additive usually derived from grain-based sources, often corn. Follow Your Heart is a good brand to try. This brand is usually sold in blocks, so you'll need to crumble or shred the cheese before using in this recipe.

4 ears corn, husked

1 tablespoon regular olive oil

Sea salt

Freshly ground black pepper

2 tablespoons unsalted butter, melted

2 tablespoons Garlic Aïoli (page 281)

¼ teaspoon paprika

¼ cup crumbled queso fresco or cotija

Juice of 1 lime

1. Prepare a gas or charcoal grill for high-heat cooking.

2. Brush the corn with the oil, and season with salt and pepper. Grill the corn, turning occasionally, for about 8 minutes, or until charred on all sides.

3. Brush with the butter and Garlic Aïoli, season with paprika, and sprinkle the queso fresco all over. Squeeze lime juice over the corn just before serving.

PER SERVING CALORIES: 233 FAT: 19 G TOTAL CARBOHYDRATES: 16 G
DIETARY FIBER: 2 G SUGARS: 3 G PROTEIN: 5 G

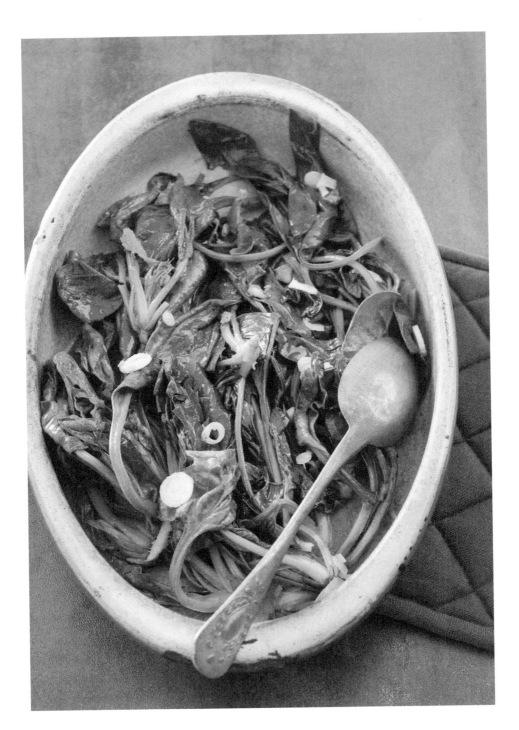

SAUTÉED SPINACH WITH NUTMEG

Dairy-Free | Nut-Free | Paleo-Friendly | Vegan

PREP TIME: 3 MINUTES ▲ COOK TIME: 6 MINUTES

SERVES 4   *Fresh spinach and a little ground nutmeg are a classic combination. If you like this side dish, try using the same preparation on Swiss chard, which has a similar flavor to spinach.*

Ingredient Variation: If you use Swiss chard, separate the stems and leaves, and cook the chopped stems first, which take longer to soften than the leaves (about 5 minutes over medium heat should do it). Then add the leaves, cooking until just wilted.

Timesaving Tip: Fresh spinach can harbor a lot of dirt, which means it needs to be washed several times. Save time by purchasing prewashed spinach, located in the refrigerated section near the salad dressings.

2 tablespoons extra-virgin olive oil

6 garlic cloves, chopped

2 bunches spinach

½ teaspoon ground nutmeg

Sea salt

Freshly ground black pepper

1. In a large pot, heat the oil over medium heat.

2. Add the garlic, and cook for 1 minute, or until golden.

3. Add the spinach, and cook for 3 to 4 minutes, or just until wilted.

4. Season with the nutmeg, salt, and pepper before serving.

PER SERVING   CALORIES: 107   FAT: 8 G   TOTAL CARBOHYDRATES: 8 G
DIETARY FIBER: 4 G   SUGARS: 1 G   PROTEIN: 5 G

SNAPPY GREEN BEANS WITH LEMON ZEST AND OLIVE TAPENADE

Dairy-Free | Nut-Free

PREP TIME: 5 MINUTES ⟁ COOK TIME: 10 MINUTES

SERVES 4   *Green beans should be cooked for just a few minutes so they're snappy, not mushy. Some lemon zest and tapenade—a Provençal paste of black olives, capers, and olive oil—goes well with the beans. Feel free to use a mixture of green and yellow beans for this dish.*

Timesaving Tip: To trim green beans quickly, line them up in a row by the stem ends, and slice off all at once. Repeat with the other side.

Sea salt

1 pound green beans, trimmed

1 tablespoon extra-virgin olive oil

3 garlic cloves, thinly sliced

Zest of 1 lemon

¼ cup Olive Tapenade (page 284)

Freshly ground black pepper

1. Bring a large pot of salted water to a boil over high heat, and fill a large bowl with ice water.

2. Add the beans to the pot and blanch the beans for 3 to 4 minutes, or until crisp-tender, and transfer with tongs to the ice water. Drain, and pat dry.

3. In a medium skillet, heat the oil over medium heat. Add the garlic, and cook for about 1 minute, or until fragrant. Add the beans, and heat through for 2 to 3 minutes, or until tender.

4. Top with the lemon zest and Olive Tapenade, and season with salt and pepper before serving.

PER SERVING CALORIES: 73 FAT: 4 G TOTAL CARBOHYDRATES: 10 G
DIETARY FIBER: 4 G SUGARS: 2 G PROTEIN: 2 G

FLUFFY MASHED CAULIFLOWER WITH THYME

Nut-Free | Paleo-Friendly

PREP TIME: 10 MINUTES ▲ COOK TIME: 10 MINUTES

SERVES 4   *Mashed cauliflower is a great alternative to mashed potatoes. You can substitute parsley, dill, or another herb for the thyme. Serve with your favorite grilled meats and poultry as a side dish.*

Diet Variation: To make this recipe dairy-free, use almond milk.

1 head cauliflower, cut into florets

1 cup nonfat milk

1 tablespoon fresh thyme leaves

Sea salt

Freshly ground black pepper

1. Bring a large pot of water to a boil over high heat.

2. Add the cauliflower, and cook for about 6 minutes, or until it is easily pierced with a fork.

3. Drain the cauliflower, and transfer to the bowl of a food processor. While the machine is running, pour in the milk. Process until combined.

4. Transfer the cauliflower mixture to a large bowl. Add the thyme, and season with salt and pepper before serving.

PER SERVING   CALORIES: 41   FAT: 0 G   TOTAL CARBOHYDRATES: 7 G
DIETARY FIBER: 2 G   SUGARS: 5 G   PROTEIN: 3 G

ROASTED SWEET POTATO FRIES WITH CUMIN, CORIANDER, AND LIME

Dairy-Free I Nut-Free I Paleo-Friendly I Vegan

PREP TIME: 5 MINUTES ▲ COOK TIME: 20 MINUTES

SERVES 4   *The smoky flavor of cumin and the bright, zesty flavor of coriander lend an exotic touch to everyone's favorite healthy alternative to French fries. Try serving them with a tasty dip, like Garlic Hummus with Tahini (page 114) for a satisfying snack.*

1 pound sweet potatoes, cut into wedges

2 tablespoons regular olive oil

Juice of 1 lime

1 teaspoon ground coriander

1 teaspoon ground cumin

Sea salt

Freshly ground black pepper

1. Preheat the oven to 450°F.

2. In a baking dish, coat the potato wedges with the oil and lime juice, and season with the coriander, cumin, salt, and pepper.

3. Roast for 20 minutes, or until the wedges are easily pierced with a fork.

PER SERVING   CALORIES: 201   FAT: 7 G   TOTAL CARBOHYDRATES: 34 G
DIETARY FIBER: 5 G   SUGARS: 1 G   PROTEIN: 2 G

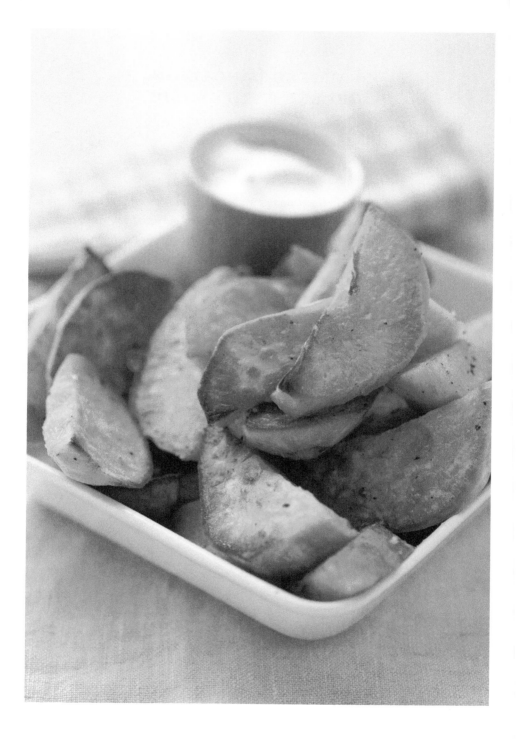

SAUTÉED DANDELION GREENS WITH GARLIC

Dairy-Free | Nut-Free | Paleo-Friendly | Vegan

PREP TIME: 3 MINUTES ▲ COOK TIME: 12 MINUTES

SERVES 4   *Dinner in Greek homes would be incomplete without a bowl of* horta, *or boiled greens, dressed with olive oil and garlic. If you can't find dandelion greens, substitute spinach or chicory. Horta goes well with rich, oily fish like sardines and anchovies, wild Alaskan salmon, Arctic char, mackerel, or steelhead trout.*

Ingredient Tip: The best time to try dandelion greens is in the spring when they are the least bitter. If picking your own, make sure they haven't been sprayed with pesticides.

2 tablespoons extra-virgin olive oil

3 garlic cloves, thinly sliced

1 bunch dandelion greens, stemmed and chopped

Sea salt

Freshly ground black pepper

1. In a large pot, heat the oil over medium heat.

2. Add the garlic, and cook for 1 minute, or until golden. Add the greens, and cook until wilted, 8 to 10 minutes. Season with salt and pepper before serving.

PER SERVING   CALORIES: 75   FAT: 7 G   TOTAL CARBOHYDRATES: 3 G
DIETARY FIBER: 1 G   SUGARS: 0 G   PROTEIN: 1 G

SAUTÉED SWISS CHARD WITH RAISINS AND ALMONDS

Dairy-Free | Vegan

PREP TIME: 5 MINUTES ▲ COOK TIME: 14 MINUTES

SERVES 4 *If you can find rainbow chard with its variously colored stems, go for it. Instead of raisins and toasted almonds, you can try different ingredient combinations such as currants and walnuts or dried figs and hazelnuts.*

Diet Variation: For a nut-free variation, substitute pomegranate seeds or pumpkin seeds for the almonds.

2 tablespoons extra-virgin olive oil

½ cup sliced raw almonds

3 garlic cloves, thinly sliced

1 bunch Swiss chard, chopped

¼ cup raisins

Sea salt

Freshly ground black pepper

1. In a large pot, heat the oil over medium heat.

2. Add the almonds, and cook for about 1½ minutes, or until toasted. Add the garlic, and cook for 1 minute, or until golden. Add the Swiss chard and raisins, and season with salt and pepper.

3. Cook for 8 to 10 minutes, or until the leaves are wilted and the stems are crisp-tender.

PER SERVING CALORIES: 187 FAT: 13 G TOTAL CARBOHYDRATES: 16 G
DIETARY FIBER: 4 G SUGARS: 8 G PROTEIN: 6 G

CABBAGE SLAW WITH BUTTERMILK DRESSING

Nut-Free | Vegetarian

PREP TIME: 10 MINUTES

SERVES 4   *Coleslaw is too often tossed with a heavy mayonnaise dressing. Using buttermilk in the dressing keeps the cabbage crisp. Try this coleslaw with the Marinated Barbecued Shrimp (page 168).*

Timesaving Tip: A food processor makes quick work of shredding cabbage. Cut the head into pieces small enough to fit into the feed tube, and use the shredding disk.

½ **head green cabbage, shredded**

1 **cup shredded carrots**

½ **cup Buttermilk Dressing (page 289)**

Sea salt

Freshly ground black pepper

1. In a large mixing bowl, toss the cabbage and carrots with the Buttermilk Dressing.

2. Season with salt and pepper.

PER SERVING   CALORIES: 222   FAT: 19 G   TOTAL CARBOHYDRATES: 14 G
DIETARY FIBER: 5 G   SUGARS: 8 G   PROTEIN: 3 G

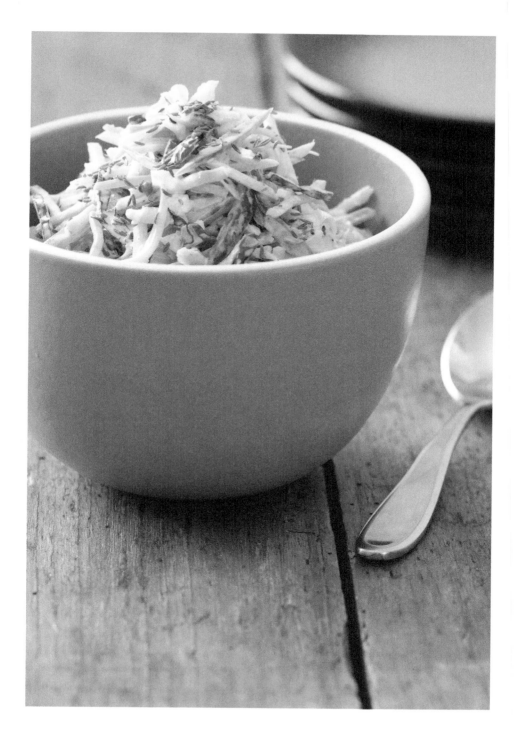

ROASTED ASPARAGUS WITH GARLIC AND ORANGE ZEST

Dairy-Free | Nut-Free | Paleo-Friendly | Vegan

PREP TIME: 10 MINUTES ▲ COOK TIME: 15 MINUTES

SERVES 4 *Local asparagus only comes around once a year during the spring. This simple side dish is one you'll want to make until asparagus runs out because it allows the clean, verdant flavor of the vegetable to shine. When choosing asparagus for this recipe, look for bunches with similar size stalks. Thinner stalks will cook more quickly.*

1 bunch asparagus, trimmed

1 tablespoon regular olive oil

3 garlic cloves, thinly sliced

Zest of 1 orange

Sea salt

Freshly ground black pepper

1. Preheat the oven to 425°F.

2. In a baking dish, coat the asparagus with the oil. Top with the garlic and orange zest. Season with salt and pepper. Roast in the oven for 12 to 15 minutes, or until the asparagus is tender and charred in spots.

PER SERVING CALORIES: 89 FAT: 4 G TOTAL CARBOHYDRATES: 13 G
DIETARY FIBER: 5 G SUGARS: 8 G PROTEIN: 4 G

ROASTED CHERRY TOMATOES WITH ARUGULA-WALNUT PESTO

Dairy-Free | Paleo-Friendly | Vegan

PREP TIME: 5 MINUTES ▲ COOK TIME: 15 MINUTES

SERVES 4   *When sweet cherry tomatoes are in season, it's hard to stop eating them like candy. Roasting cherry tomatoes brings out their natural sweetness, and when complemented with slightly piquant Arugula-Walnut Pesto, they become a side to serve with grilled fish, poultry, or meats.*

> 1 pound mixed ripe cherry tomatoes
> 2 tablespoons regular olive oil
> Sea salt
> Freshly ground black pepper
> ¼ cup Arugula-Walnut Pesto (page 275)

1. Preheat the oven to 400°F.

2. In a baking dish, coat the tomatoes with oil, and season with salt and pepper. Roast in the oven for 15 minutes, or until soft and blistered.

3. Remove from the oven, and serve with the Arugula-Walnut Pesto on top.

PER SERVING   CALORIES: 147   FAT: 14 G   TOTAL CARBOHYDRATES: 5 G
DIETARY FIBER: 2 G   SUGARS: 3 G   PROTEIN: 3 G

SOUTHERN-STYLE COLLARD GREENS WITH SMOKED BACON

Dairy-Free | Nut-Free

PREP TIME: 4 MINUTES ▲ COOK TIME: 41 MINUTES

SERVES 4   *These collard greens are tender and have a hint of sweetness. Choose bunches with bright green, intact leaves, and cut off the tough stems before cooking the collards. If you like things on the spicy side, serve with some hot sauce. These go well with anything that comes off a grill.*

¼ pound smoked bacon, chopped

3 garlic cloves

1 bunch collard greens, stemmed and chopped

Sea salt

Cayenne pepper

2 cups vegetable stock

1 tablespoon distilled white vinegar or apple cider vinegar

1 tablespoon honey

Dash hot sauce (optional)

1. In a large pot, cook the bacon over medium heat for 5 minutes, or until the fat is rendered and the bacon is crisp.

2. Add the garlic, and cook for 1 minute, or until golden. Add the collard greens, season with salt and cayenne pepper, and cook for 5 minutes.

3. Add the stock, vinegar, honey, and hot sauce (if using), and bring to a simmer. Simmer for about 30 minutes, or until the collard greens are tender.

PER SERVING   CALORIES: 219   FAT: 13 G   TOTAL CARBOHYDRATES: 14 G
DIETARY FIBER: 5 G   SUGARS: 5 G   PROTEIN: 14 G

RED WINE–BRAISED
RED CABBAGE

Dairy-Free | Nut-Free | Vegan

SERVES 4   *The wine infuses the cabbage as it cooks slowly over the stove and turns it tender at the same time. Serve it with dishes that feature smoky meats like Hearty Sausage and Bean Stew (page 221).*

½ **bottle red wine**

2 cups vegetable stock

1 head red cabbage, shredded

3 garlic cloves, smashed

Sea salt

Freshly ground black pepper

1. In a large pot, bring the wine and stock to a simmer.

2. Add the cabbage and garlic, and season with salt and pepper.

3. Simmer, covered, for about 30 minutes, or until the cabbage is tender.

PER SERVING   CALORIES: 134   FAT: 0 G   TOTAL CARBOHYDRATES: 15 G
DIETARY FIBER: 5 G   SUGARS: 7 G   PROTEIN: 3 G

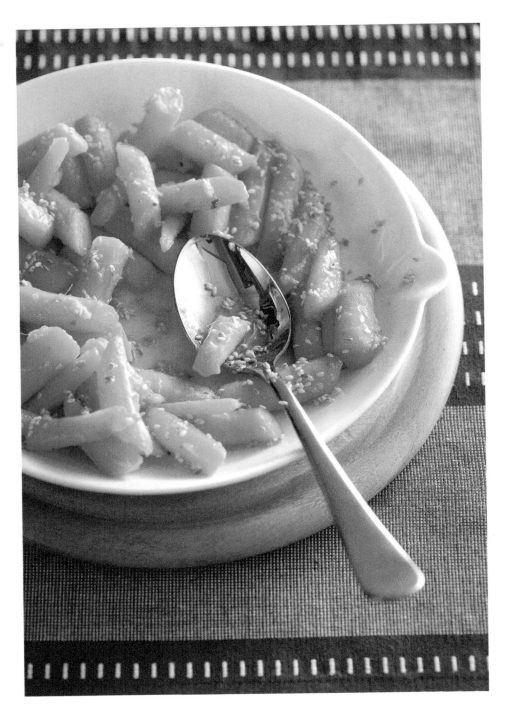

HONEY-ROASTED CARROTS

Dairy-Free | Nut-Free | Paleo-Friendly | Vegetarian

PREP TIME: 5 MINUTES ▲ COOK TIME: 20 MINUTES

SERVES 4   *These carrots are sweet and tangy with just a hit of spiciness—a winning combination. They are brushed with honey and tossed with sesame seeds and a bit of lime juice before going into the oven. Pair with chicken, pork, beef, or lamb dishes. The baby carrots used in this recipe aren't the precut ones. Instead, look for small carrots that come in bunches with the green tops intact.*

1 pound baby carrots

1 tablespoon honey

1 tablespoon regular olive oil

1 teaspoon white sesame seeds

Juice of 1 lime

1 teaspoon ground cumin

1 teaspoon ground coriander

Sea salt

Freshly ground black pepper

1. Preheat the oven to 400°F.

2. In a baking dish, toss the carrots with the honey, oil, sesame seeds, and lime juice.

3. Season with the cumin, coriander, salt, and pepper. Roast the carrots for about 20 minutes, or until tender.

PER SERVING   CALORIES: 96   FAT: 4 G   TOTAL CARBOHYDRATES: 16 G
DIETARY FIBER: 4 G   SUGARS: 10 G   PROTEIN: 1 G

PAN-ROASTED BRUSSELS SPROUTS WITH RED PEPPER FLAKES AND PARMESAN

Nut-Free | Vegetarian

PREP TIME: 5 MINUTES ▲ COOK TIME: 40 MINUTES

SERVES 4   *Until recently, no one much cared for Brussels sprouts because the mini-cabbages were usually boiled to death. Pan-roasting Brussels sprouts brings out their inherent sweetness. The key is to cut them in half, getting the interiors nice and tender and the cut sides nice and browned. A light dusting of Parmesan at the end enhances their natural nutty flavor, but you can try other hard cheeses like pecorino or manchego.*

Diet Variation: To make this recipe vegan, substitute chopped sun-dried tomatoes or toasted pine nuts for the Parmesan.

2 tablespoons regular olive oil

1 pound Brussels sprouts, halved

1 teaspoon red pepper flakes

Sea salt

Freshly ground black pepper

¼ cup grated Parmesan

1. Preheat the oven to 400°F.

2. Heat the oil in an ovenproof skillet over medium-high heat.

3. Place the Brussels sprouts cut side down, and sauté for about 3 to 5 minutes, or until browned on the bottom. Shake the pan, season with the red pepper flakes and salt and pepper, and transfer to the oven. Roast for about 35 minutes, or until the Brussels sprouts are easily pierced with a fork.

4. Sprinkle on the Parmesan just before serving.

PER SERVING   CALORIES: 128   FAT: 9 G   TOTAL CARBOHYDRATES: 11 G
DIETARY FIBER: 4 G   SUGARS: 3 G   PROTEIN: 6 G

ROASTED ROSEMARY POTATOES

Dairy-Free | Nut-Free | Vegan

PREP TIME: 5 MINUTES ▲ COOK TIME: 40 MINUTES

SERVES 4   *The secret to great roasted potatoes is to add fresh herbs and lots of garlic. These roasted spuds certainly don't skimp on either of those things. Choose smaller potatoes or cut the potatoes into smaller pieces to reduce cooking time. While Yukon Gold potatoes are used here, feel free to experiment with other waxy or semi-waxy potatoes.*

Cooking Tip: When it comes to cutting potatoes, the more edges you give them, the crunchier they will be on the outside.

- 1 pound Yukon Gold potatoes, cut into bite-size pieces
- 2 tablespoons regular olive oil
- 3 garlic cloves, thinly sliced
- 1 tablespoon chopped fresh rosemary
- Sea salt
- Freshly ground black pepper

1. Preheat the oven to 475°F.

2. In a medium bowl, toss the potatoes with the oil, garlic, and rosemary. Season with salt and pepper.

3. Transfer to a baking dish, and roast for 40 minutes, or until the potatoes are easily pierced with a fork.

PER SERVING   CALORIES: 150   FAT: 7 G   TOTAL CARBOHYDRATES: 21 G
DIETARY FIBER: 2 G   SUGARS: 1 G   PROTEIN: 3 G

CHAPTER 8

Vegetarian and Vegan

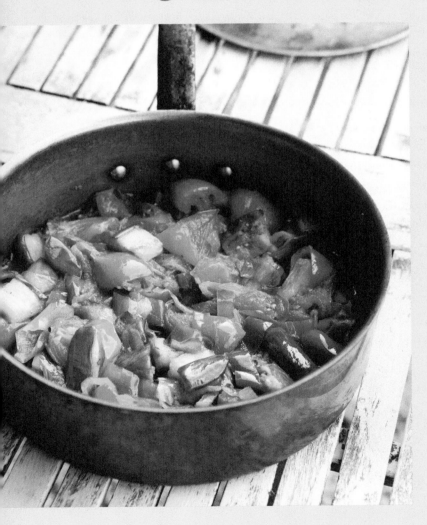

PEACH, FETA, AND MINT CAPRESE SALAD

Nut-Free | Vegetarian

PREP TIME: 5 MINUTES

SERVES 4 *While a Caprese salad is traditionally made with tomatoes, moz-zarella, and basil, experiment with other fruits, cheeses, and herbs. Another combination that's equally delicious is pineapple, queso fresco, and cilantro.*

Ingredient Tip: Did you know that there are two main types of peaches? A clingstone peach has a pit that "clings" stubbornly to the flesh, no matter how ripe it is. Freestone peaches have a pit that is easily removed when the fruit is ripe. Generally speaking, if you're buying your peaches at the supermarket, they'll be freestone. So if the two halves of the peach don't twist easily around the pit when you slice around the middle, then the peach isn't ripe.

1 pound ripe peaches
Sea salt
Freshly ground black pepper
¼ pound crumbled feta
½ cup mint leaves
¼ cup extra-virgin olive oil

1. Hold 1 peach in one hand, and rotate it while tracing a line all the way through to the pit using a chef's knife.

2. Twist the two halves apart, remove the pit, and slice thinly. Repeat for the remaining peaches, and season the peach slices with salt and pepper.

3. Divide the peach slices among 4 plates, and top with the feta and mint leaves. Drizzle the oil on top before serving.

PER SERVING   CALORIES: 232   FAT: 19 G   TOTAL CARBOHYDRATES: 13 G
DIETARY FIBER: 3 G   SUGARS: 11 G   PROTEIN: 5 G

ARUGULA SALAD WITH RADISHES, POMEGRANATE SEEDS, AND PINE NUTS

Dairy-Free | Paleo-Friendly | Vegan

PREP TIME: 10 MINUTES

SERVES 4   *There's certainly plenty of crunch in this salad, with thinly sliced radishes, a handful of pomegranate seeds, and toasted pine nuts. Toasting pine nuts accentuates their rich flavor and only takes a few minutes, and pomegranate seeds add a nice fruity touch to balance out the flavors of this salad. Serve as a light lunch or a fantastic starter for dinner.*

....

Ingredient Tip: To get the seeds out of a pomegranate, cut the fruit into four to six wedges, and hold each wedge cut side down over a large bowl. Whack each wedge with the back of a wooden spoon, and the seeds will fall right out.

....

Note: To toast the pine nuts, place them in a skillet over medium-low heat, shaking occasionally, for about 3 minutes, or until they are golden brown. Watch carefully, as they can start to burn in seconds.

- 1 bunch arugula
- 1 bunch red radishes, thinly sliced
- ½ cup pomegranate seeds
- ¼ cup pine nuts, toasted
- ¼ cup Lemon Vinaigrette (page 286)
- Sea salt
- Freshly ground black pepper

1. In a large mixing bowl, toss the arugula, radishes, pomegranate seeds, and pine nuts with the Lemon Vinaigrette.

2. Season with salt and pepper.

PER SERVING   CALORIES: 162   FAT: 16 G   TOTAL CARBOHYDRATES: 6 G
DIETARY FIBER: 1 G   SUGARS: 3 G   PROTEIN: 2 G

HEIRLOOM TOMATO
CAPRESE SALAD

Nut-Free | Vegetarian

PREP TIME: 5 MINUTES

SERVES 4   *Heirloom tomatoes are grown from seeds that have been passed down through several generations. Like other tomatoes, they come in all different shapes, colors, and sizes. One of the simplest ways to showcase their variety is to pair them with thin slices of fresh mozzarella. For an interesting variation, try buffalo mozzarella, which has a creamier texture and richer flavor than mozzarella made from cow's milk.*

Ingredient Tip: Season the tomatoes with salt just before serving them. If you salt them too far in advance, they will become soggy.

1 pound heirloom tomatoes, thinly sliced

½ pound fresh mozzarella, thinly sliced

Sea salt

Freshly ground black pepper

1 cup basil leaves

¼ cup extra-virgin olive oil

1. Season the tomato and mozzarella slices with salt and pepper.

2. Set out 4 plates. Divide the heirloom tomato and mozzarella slices among the plates, alternating layers.

3. Top with the basil. Drizzle the oil on top before serving.

PER SERVING   CALORIES: 292   FAT: 23 G   TOTAL CARBOHYDRATES: 7 G
DIETARY FIBER: 2 G   SUGARS: 3 G   PROTEIN: 17 G

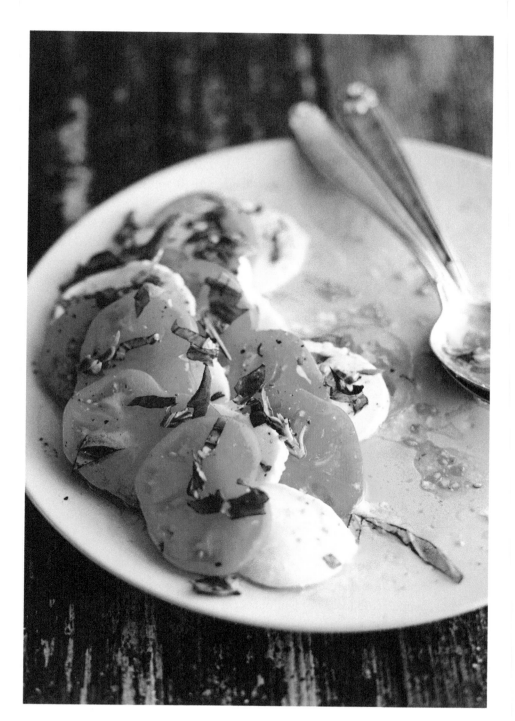

GRILLED PORTOBELLO MUSHROOMS WITH CHARMOULA

Dairy-Free | Nut-Free | Paleo-Friendly | Vegan

PREP TIME: 5 MINUTES ▲ COOK TIME: 10 MINUTES

SERVES 4   *Charmoula, a cilantro-based Moroccan condiment, adds zestiness to grilled portobello mushrooms. Prepare the Charmoula (page 283) as the grill preheats, which will leave you time to prepare a quick side as the mushrooms are cooking. This is a complete meal that can hit the dinner table in very little time. If you're looking for a great side dish to go with this vegetarian main course, you may want to try the Honey-Roasted Carrots (page 133), whose flavors complement Charmoula nicely. For a great starter, try the Creamy Charred Eggplant Dip (page 88) and serve with your favorite chopped fresh vegetables for dipping.*

Ingredient Tip: When grilling portobello mushrooms, choose ones with flatter caps, which will cook more uniformly on the grill.

4 portobello mushrooms, stemmed

¼ cup regular olive oil

Sea salt

Freshly ground black pepper

½ cup Charmoula (page 283)

1. Prepare a gas or charcoal grill for high-heat cooking.

2. Brush the mushrooms with the oil, and season with salt and pepper. Grill for about 5 minutes per side, or until the mushrooms are tender and easily pierced with a fork in the center.

3. Serve the mushrooms with the Charmoula on top.

PER SERVING   CALORIES: 285   FAT: 30 G   TOTAL CARBOHYDRATES: 4 G
DIETARY FIBER: 1 G   SUGARS: 0 G   PROTEIN: 3 G

QUICK RATATOUILLE AND QUINOA

Dairy-Free | Nut-Free | Paleo-Friendly | Vegan

PREP TIME: 15 MINUTES ▲ COOK TIME: 15 MINUTES

SERVES 4   *Ratatouille, a Provençal summer vegetable dish from southern France, usually takes a fair amount of time to make. This recipe simplifies the process by cooking all of the vegetables at the same time in the oven, turning it into a practical weeknight meal. Served over a bed of quinoa, this dish becomes a great source of protein. If there are any leftovers, they can easily be reheated for lunch the next day.*

¼ cup extra-virgin olive oil

5 garlic cloves, chopped

1 pound zucchini, chopped

2 ripe beefsteak tomatoes, chopped

1 pound eggplants, chopped

3 red bell peppers, stemmed, seeded, and chopped

Sea salt

Freshly ground black pepper

¼ cup chopped fresh tarragon

¼ cup chopped fresh oregano

2 tablespoons chopped fresh thyme

2 cups water

1 cup quinoa

1. Preheat the oven to 500°F.

2. In a large baking dish, mix the oil, garlic, zucchini, tomatoes, eggplant, and bell peppers. Season with salt and pepper, and top with the tarragon, oregano, and thyme. Roast in the oven for about 15 minutes, or until the vegetables are tender. »

3. Meanwhile, in a medium pot, bring the water, lightly salted, to a boil. Add the quinoa, reduce the heat to a simmer, cover, and cook for about 12 minutes, or until all of the water is absorbed and the hard white center of each seed is no longer visible.

4. Serve the quinoa topped with the hot ratatouille.

PER SERVING   CALORIES: 368   FAT: 17 G   TOTAL CARBOHYDRATES: 50 G
DIETARY FIBER: 13 G   SUGARS: 10 G   PROTEIN: 11 G

VEGETABLE BEAN SOUP

Dairy-Free | Nut-Free | Vegan

PREP TIME: 10 MINUTES ▲ COOK TIME: 30 MINUTES

SERVES 8   *Vegetable bean soup is hearty and satisfying without being too heavy. It's perfect for lunch or dinner on a winter's day. This recipe calls for cannellini beans, but you can substitute kidney, navy, or black beans.*

- 2 tablespoons extra-virgin olive oil
- 3 garlic cloves
- 1 red onion, chopped
- 2 carrots, chopped
- 2 celery stalks, chopped
- Sea salt
- Freshly ground black pepper
- 1 tablespoon tomato paste
- 2 quarts (8 cups) vegetable stock
- 1 bunch lacinato kale, leaves removed from stems and chopped
- 1 pound baby red potatoes, quartered
- 2 (15-ounce) cans cannellini beans, drained and rinsed

1. In a large pot, heat the oil over medium heat.

2. Add the garlic, onion, carrots, and celery; season with salt and pepper; and cook for 10 to 15 minutes, or until softened. Make room in the center, add the tomato paste, and cook for 1 minute. Add the stock, cover, bring to a simmer, and add the kale and potatoes. Simmer for 8 to 10 minutes, or until the potatoes are nearly fork tender.

3. Add the beans, and simmer for 2 to 3 minutes, or until softened and slightly creamy.

PER SERVING   CALORIES: 482   FAT: 5 G   TOTAL CARBOHYDRATES: 84 G
DIETARY FIBER: 31 G   SUGARS: 6 G   PROTEIN: 29 G

GAZPACHO

Dairy-Free | Nut-Free | Paleo-Friendly | Vegan

SERVES 4   *Gazpacho, a chilled soup from Andalusia in southern Spain, is most frequently made with tomatoes, cucumbers, and peppers, but there are many variations. If you've never made gazpacho before, this is the recipe to start with because it only takes minutes to prepare.*

Ingredient Variation: If tomatoes are not in season, try using high-quality canned whole peeled tomatoes.

- 1½ pounds ripe tomatoes, sliced
- 1 cucumber, peeled, seeded, and roughly chopped
- 1 red bell pepper, stemmed, seeded, and roughly chopped
- 1 green bell pepper, stemmed, seeded, and roughly chopped
- 2 tablespoons extra-virgin olive oil
- 1 tablespoon sherry vinegar
- 1 teaspoon paprika
- Sea salt
- Freshly ground black pepper

1. In a blender or the bowl of a food processor, add the tomatoes, cucumber, green and red bell peppers (reserving some for garnish, if desired), oil, vinegar, and paprika.

2. Season with salt and pepper.

3. Process until smooth, and chill in the refrigerator before serving. Garnish with the reserved vegetables, if using.

PER SERVING CALORIES: 122 FAT: 8 G TOTAL CARBOHYDRATES: 13 G
DIETARY FIBER: 4 G SUGARS: 7 G PROTEIN: 3 G

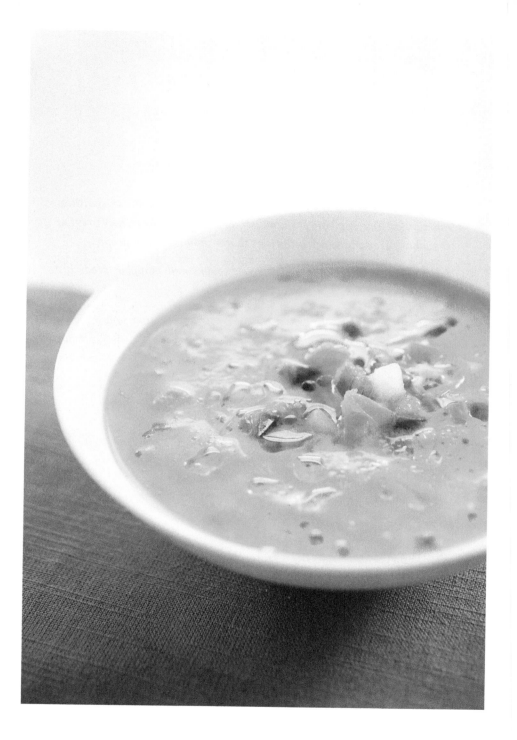

BUTTERNUT SQUASH SOUP WITH SAGE

Dairy-Free I Nut-Free I Paleo-Friendly I Vegan

PREP TIME: 5 MINUTES ▲ COOK TIME: 40 MINUTES

SERVES 4   *Butternut squash soup has become an American tradition, especially at Thanksgiving or the winter holidays. You'll learn how to cut up the squash properly, which is the part that intimidates most people.*

Ingredient Variation: Add some Greek yogurt and pumpkin seeds just before serving to add some tanginess and crunch.

Timesaving Tip: You can purchase peeled, cut-up butternut squash, found next to the prepackaged salads in the refrigerated section of the supermarket. You'll need about 2½ to 3 cups cubed. If you're using precut squash, skip the first five steps in the instructions.

1 (2-pound) butternut squash
2 tablespoons regular olive oil
Sea salt
Freshly ground black pepper
1 quart (4 cups) vegetable stock
2 tablespoons finely chopped fresh sage

1. Preheat the oven to 475°F.

2. Using the base of a chef's knife, cut off the stem at the top of the squash.

3. Using a vegetable peeler, peel the skin from the squash.

4. Using a knife, cut the squash into quarters.

5. Using a spoon, scoop out the seeds.

6. Chop the squash into small chunks, transfer to a baking sheet, coat with the oil, and season with salt and pepper.

7. Roast in the oven for about 40 minutes, or until tender.

8. Transfer to a blender or the bowl of a food processor together with the stock, and process until smooth. Serve topped with sage.

PER SERVING   CALORIES: 205   FAT: 8 G   TOTAL CARBOHYDRATES: 36 G
DIETARY FIBER: 7 G   SUGARS: 8 G   PROTEIN: 4 G

CREAMY CORN CHOWDER

Nut-Free | Vegetarian

PREP TIME: 10 MINUTES ▲ COOK TIME: 35 MINUTES

SERVES 4   *Fresh sweet corn is the key to this summery vegetarian starter. Choose corn that is still in the husk with moist threads and brightly colored leaves. Squeeze a kernel gently to see if it releases some juice—this is another sign of freshness. Serve this with Marinated Barbecued Shrimp (page 168) or some Steamed Mussels with Parsley, Lemon, and Shallot (page 173).*

Diet Variation: To make a dairy-free version of this recipe, substitute 2 cups of almond milk for the nonfat milk.

4 ears corn, husked

2 tablespoons extra-virgin olive oil

3 garlic cloves, chopped

1 red onion, finely chopped

1 cup vegetable stock

2 cups nonfat milk

½ pound baby red potatoes, finely diced

Sea salt

Freshly ground black pepper

1. Remove the kernels from the corn by placing the flat end of each ear on a firm surface and slicing down each side with a chef's knife.

2. In a medium pot, heat the oil over medium heat. Add the garlic and onion, and cook for 5 to 7 minutes, or until the onion is crisp-tender. Add the corn, and cook for 5 to 7 minutes, or until crisp-tender. Add the stock, milk, and potatoes, and bring the mixture to a simmer. Cook for 8 to 10 minutes, or until the potatoes are tender.

3. Transfer 2 cups of the soup to a blender or the bowl of a food processor, and process until smooth.

4. Add the mixture back to the soup, and simmer for 5 to 10 minutes, or until thickened. Season with salt and pepper before serving.

PER SERVING   CALORIES: 222   FAT: 8 G   TOTAL CARBOHYDRATES: 33 G
DIETARY FIBER: 4 G   SUGARS: 11 G   PROTEIN: 8 G

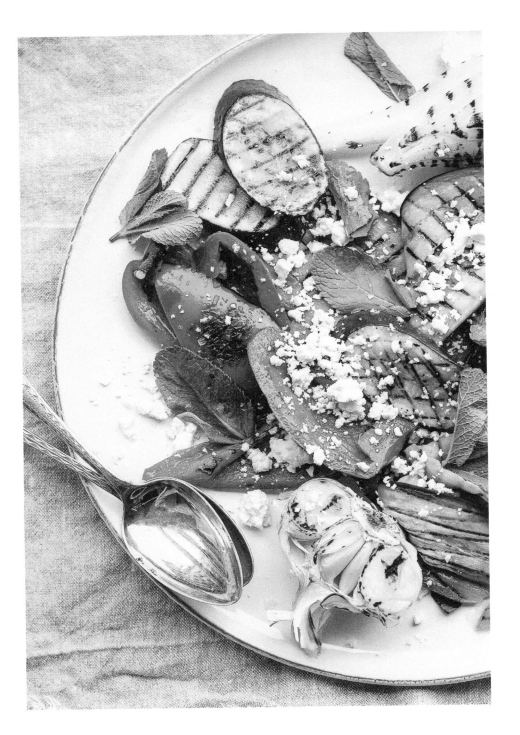

GRILLED ZUCCHINI AND EGGPLANT SALAD WITH FETA AND RED ONION

Nut-Free | Vegetarian

PREP TIME: 5 MINUTES ▲ COOK TIME: 10 MINUTES

SERVES 4   *This starter is a celebration of summer with its vibrant colors and simple preparation. Drizzle with a refreshing Lemon Vinaigrette and serve it with grilled meats or seafood. When choosing zucchini, opt for the smaller ones, which are tastier.*

Diet Variation: To make this dish dairy-free, substitute toasted almonds or pine nuts for the feta.

½ pound zucchini, cut into ¼-inch-thick slices lengthwise

½ pound eggplant, cut into ¼-inch-thick slices lengthwise

1 red bell pepper, stemmed, seeded, and cut into wedges

½ head garlic

2 tablespoons regular olive oil

Sea salt

Freshly ground black pepper

¼ pound crumbled feta

½ red onion, thinly sliced

¼ cup mint leaves

3 tablespoons Lemon Vinaigrette (page 286)

1. Prepare a gas or charcoal grill for medium-high-heat cooking.

2. Coat the zucchini, eggplant, bell pepper, and garlic with the oil, and season with salt and pepper. Grill for 2 to 4 minutes per side, or until grill marks appear.

3. Transfer to a platter, and top with the feta, red onion, and mint leaves. Drizzle the Lemon Vinaigrette on top before serving.

PER SERVING CALORIES: 37 FAT: 21 G TOTAL CARBOHYDRATES: 10 G
DIETARY FIBER: 4 G SUGARS: 4 G PROTEIN: 6 G

VEGETARIAN CHILES RELLENOS WITH TOASTED WALNUTS, RAISINS, AND MONTEREY JACK

Vegetarian

PREP TIME: 10 MINUTES ▲ COOK TIME: 30 MINUTES

SERVES 4 *In these vegetarian chiles rellenos, toasted walnuts replace the traditional ground meat, raisins add a burst of sweetness, and Monterey Jack cheese melts into the other ingredients as the dish browns in the oven. If you can't find the poblano peppers called for in this recipe, bell peppers can be used as a substitute.*

Timesaving Tip: This technique of charring peppers directly over a flame can be applied to any pepper, enhancing its flavor. Placing them in a bag once charred will allow them to steam, making it easier to remove the skin.

- 4 poblano peppers
- 2 tablespoons regular olive oil
- 1½ teaspoons ground cumin
- Sea salt
- Freshly ground black pepper
- 1 cup walnuts, toasted and finely chopped
- 1 cup raisins
- ¼ pound Monterey Jack cheese, shredded

1. Place the peppers directly over a gas flame for about 15 minutes, rotating occasionally, or until charred and blackened all over. Transfer to a paper bag for about 10 minutes, slip the skins off, and cut a slit down the middle.

2. Preheat the oven to 350°F.

3. Coat the peppers with the oil, and season with the cumin, salt, and pepper. Stuff the peppers with the walnuts and raisins, and top with the cheese.

4. Place upright in a small baking dish or ovenproof pan, and roast for about 15 minutes, or until they are blistered and the cheese is melted.

PER SERVING   CALORIES: 488   FAT: 35 G   TOTAL CARBOHYDRATES: 37 G
DIETARY FIBER: 4 G   SUGARS: 24 G   PROTEIN: 17 G

ZUCCHINI AND YELLOW SQUASH PASTA WITH TOASTED HAZELNUTS AND LEMON VINAIGRETTE

Vegetarian

PREP TIME: 10 MINUTES

SERVES 4 *By using a vegetable peeler (or mandoline), you can turn zucchini and yellow squash into beautiful long ribbons. Dress them with a light Lemon Vinaigrette and toss them with toasted hazelnuts.*

Diet Variation: To make a nut-free version of this dish, substitute pomegranate seeds for the toasted hazelnuts.

- ½ pound zucchini
- ½ pound yellow squash
- 3 tablespoons Lemon Vinaigrette (page 286)
- Sea salt
- Freshly ground black pepper
- ½ cup skinned hazelnuts, toasted
- ½ cup mint leaves

1. Using a vegetable peeler, shave the zucchini and yellow squash over a medium bowl using long, continuous strokes to create ribbons.

2. Toss with the Lemon Vinaigrette, and season with salt and pepper.

3. Serve topped with hazelnuts and mint leaves.

PER SERVING CALORIES: 142 FAT: 13 G TOTAL CARBOHYDRATES: 6 G
DIETARY FIBER: 3 G SUGARS: 3 G PROTEIN: 3 G

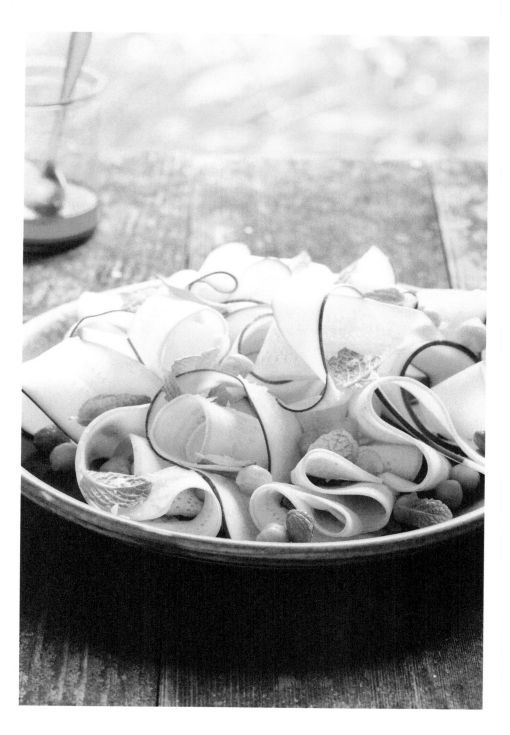

MINESTRONE ALLA GENOVESE

Vegetarian

PREP TIME: 15 MINUTES ▲ COOK TIME: 25 MINUTES

SERVES 8   *This soup is thick with green beans, chickpeas, white beans, and zucchini. The name of the dish is a reference to Genoa, the capital of Liguria, Italy, where pesto originated. Some pesto is stirred into the soup just before serving to add another layer of flavor.*

Timesaving Tip: Make quick work of peeling small amounts of garlic. Hold the flat side of your chef's knife firmly over each clove, and give the blade a firm whack with the palm of your hand. The clove should slip right out of the skin.

- 2 tablespoons extra-virgin olive oil
- 1 red onion, finely chopped
- 3 garlic cloves, thinly sliced
- Sea salt
- Freshly ground black pepper
- 2 quarts (8 cups) vegetable broth
- ½ pound zucchini, diced
- ½ pound green beans, trimmed and chopped
- 1 (15-ounce) can cannellini beans, drained and rinsed
- 1 (15-ounce) can chickpeas, drained and rinsed
- ½ cup Simple Basil Pesto (page 274)

1. In a large pot, heat the oil over medium heat.

2. Add the onion and garlic, and cook for 5 to 7 minutes, or until crisp-tender. Season with salt and pepper. Add the broth, and bring to a simmer. Add the zucchini, and cook for about 5 minutes, or until crisp-tender. Add the green beans, and cook for about 8 minutes, or until crisp-tender. Add the cannellini beans and chickpeas, and cook for 2 to 3 minutes, or until softened.

3. Divide the soup among 8 bowls. Serve the Simple Basil Pesto on top of the soup.

PER SERVING   CALORIES: 510   FAT: 14 G   TOTAL CARBOHYDRATES: 70 G
DIETARY FIBER: 24 G   SUGARS: 9 G   PROTEIN: 29 G

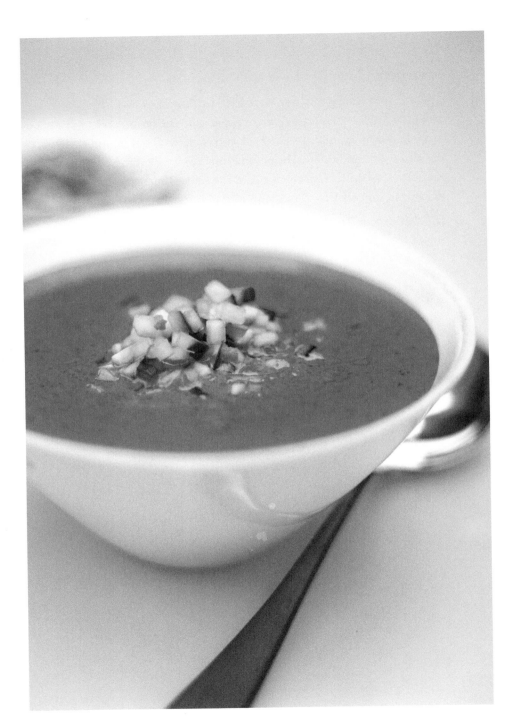

VEGETARIAN BORSCHT

Nut-Free | Vegetarian

PREP TIME: 15 MINUTES ▲ COOK TIME: 30 MINUTES

SERVES 4   *Borscht is an Eastern European soup of beets, chicken stock, carrots, and dill, often served with a bit of sour cream. In this vegetarian version, vegetable stock replaces the chicken stock and Greek yogurt takes the place of sour cream.*

2 tablespoons extra-virgin olive oil

1 red onion, chopped

1 pound red beets, peeled and grated

½ pound baby red potatoes, finely diced

2 quarts (8 cups) vegetable stock

Sea salt

Freshly ground black pepper

¼ cup chopped fresh dill

1 cup nonfat plain Greek yogurt

½ cup finely chopped cucumber, for garnish (optional)

½ cup finely chopped yellow onion, for garnish (optional)

1. In a large pot, heat the oil over medium heat.

2. Add the onion, and cook for 5 to 7 minutes, or until crisp-tender. Add the beets and potatoes, and cover with the stock.

3. Bring to a boil, reduce to a vigorous simmer, and cook for 20 minutes, or until soft enough to blend.

4. Transfer to a blender or the bowl of a food processor, and process until smooth. Season with salt and pepper.

5. Divide the soup among 4 bowls and top with the dill and Greek yogurt before serving. Garnish with the cucumber and onions (if using).

PER SERVING   CALORIES: 227 FAT: 8 G   TOTAL CARBOHYDRATES: 34 G
DIETARY FIBER: 8 G   SUGARS: 18 G   PROTEIN: 9 G

VEGETARIAN STUFFED CABBAGE

Vegetarian

PREP TIME: 20 MINUTES ▲ COOK TIME: 20 MINUTES

SERVES 4   *This Eastern European staple is usually made with a meat filling and served either with a creamy mushroom sauce or tomato sauce. This version, however, uses sautéed mushrooms, feta, and toasted walnuts for a vegetarian-friendly filling. It's a comfort food that will definitely stick to your ribs without adding to your waistline.*

1 head green cabbage, cored

¼ cup regular olive oil

2 pounds white or cremini mushrooms, chopped

Sea salt

Freshly ground black pepper

½ pound crumbled feta

½ cup finely chopped fresh flat-leaf parsley

1 cup walnuts, toasted and finely chopped

1 cup Quick Marinara Sauce (page 272)

1. Bring a large pot of salted water to a boil over high heat.

2. Boil the cabbage for 3 to 5 minutes, or until the leaves are soft enough to bend without tearing. Remove and let cool. Gently pry off the outer leaves; reserve the small inner ones for another use.

3. Meanwhile, in a large skillet, heat the oil over medium-high heat. Add the mushrooms, and cook for 10 to 15 minutes, or until golden brown. Season with salt and pepper, top with the feta and parsley, mix in the walnuts, and cover.

4. When the cabbage leaves are cool enough to handle, stuff each cabbage leaf in the center with ⅓ cup of the filling and roll, tucking the outer edges underneath.

5. Heat the Quick Marinara Sauce in a saucepan over medium heat. Spoon the sauce over the cabbage rolls before serving.

PER SERVING   CALORIES: 613   FAT: 47 G   TOTAL CARBOHYDRATES: 31 G
DIETARY FIBER: 10 G   SUGARS: 16 G   PROTEIN: 25 G

CHAPTER 9

Fish and Seafood

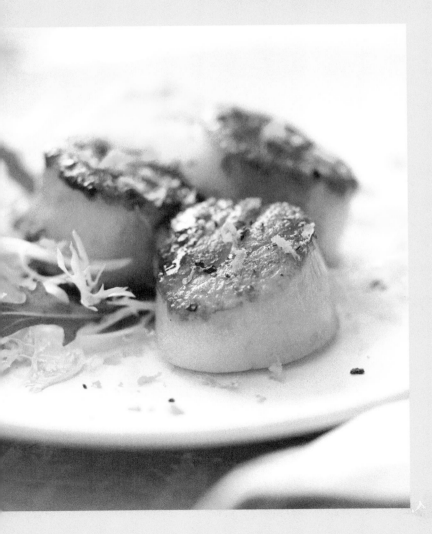

SEARED SCALLOPS WITH LEMON-HERB VINAIGRETTE

Dairy-Free | Nut-Free | Paleo-Friendly

PREP TIME: 5 MINUTES ▲ COOK TIME: 5 MINUTES

SERVES 4 *The key to searing scallops with a brown crust is to buy dry-packed sea scallops. Make sure to specifically ask for them at the seafood counter because scallops are often packed in a preservative that causes them to release liquid when cooking.*

Cooking Tip: When searing seafood, avoid seasoning with salt too far in advance. Salt draws out moisture and causes it to steam rather than sear. Instead, season seafood right before it hits the pan.

2 tablespoons regular olive oil

1 pound dry-packed sea scallops

Sea salt

Freshly ground black pepper

2 tablespoons Lemon Vinaigrette (page 286)

2 tablespoons finely chopped fresh flat-leaf parsley

Zest of ½ lemon, for garnish (optional)

1. In a large skillet, heat the oil over high heat until it is almost smoking.

2. Season the scallops with salt and pepper.

3. Place the scallops in a single layer in the pan, and cook, undisturbed, for 1½ minutes, or until a brown crust forms. Using a pair of tongs, gently turn the scallops, and cook for 1½ minutes, or just before they are cooked through. (If the scallops do not release easily, cook a little longer, and shake the pan to loosen them.)

4. Transfer with tongs to plates, drizzle with the Lemon Vinaigrette, and top with the parsley and lemon zest (if using) before serving.

PER SERVING CALORIES: 201 FAT: 13 G TOTAL CARBOHYDRATES: 3 G
DIETARY FIBER: 0 G SUGARS: 0 G PROTEIN: 19 G

PAN-SEARED SHRIMP WITH ARUGULA-WALNUT PESTO

Paleo-Friendly

PREP TIME: 5 MINUTES ▲ COOK TIME: 5 MINUTES

SERVES 4   *The pesto that most people are familiar with is made with basil, Parmesan cheese, and pine nuts. This one uses spicy arugula, toasted walnuts, and sheep's milk pecorino. Serve this with some Pan-Roasted Brussels Sprouts with Red Pepper Flakes and Parmesan (page 134) for a complete meal.*

> **2 tablespoons regular olive oil**
>
> **1 pound large shrimp, peeled and deveined**
>
> **Sea salt**
>
> **Freshly ground black pepper**
>
> **¼ cup Arugula-Walnut Pesto (page 275)**

1. In a large skillet, heat the oil over medium-high heat.

2. Season the shrimp with salt and pepper, and cook for 1 to 1½ minutes per side, or just until opaque.

3. In a medium bowl, toss the shrimp with the Arugula-Walnut Pesto, and divide them among 4 plates.

PER SERVING   CALORIES: 218   FAT: 14 G   TOTAL CARBOHYDRATES: 3 G
DIETARY FIBER: 0 G   SUGARS: 0 G   PROTEIN: 23 G

MARINATED BARBECUED SHRIMP

Dairy-Free | Nut-Free | Paleo-Friendly

PREP TIME: 5 MINUTES (PLUS MARINATING TIME) ▲ COOK TIME: 5 MINUTES

SERVES 4   *Succulent jumbo shrimp, skewered and grilled, are a great source of protein and low in fat. This recipe is simple to prepare and takes almost no time. Serve with a quick side like Roasted Asparagus with Garlic and Orange Zest (page 128) for an easy dinner.*

Timesaving Tip: To save on prep time, ask for peeled, deveined shrimp at the seafood counter. It may be a little more expensive, but it's definitely worth it.

1 pound large shrimp, peeled and deveined

1 teaspoon cayenne pepper

1 teaspoon paprika

2 tablespoons regular olive oil

Juice of 2 lemons

Sea salt

Freshly ground black pepper

¼ cup finely chopped parsley, for garnish (optional)

1. Season the shrimp with the cayenne pepper and paprika, and place in a zipper-close bag. Add the oil and lemon juice, shake to combine, and marinate for about 10 minutes.

2. Meanwhile, prepare a gas or charcoal grill for medium-heat cooking.

3. Season the shrimp with salt and pepper, and grill for 2 to 3 minutes per side, or just until cooked through. Garnish with the parsley (if using).

PER SERVING   CALORIES: 163   FAT: 7 G   TOTAL CARBOHYDRATES: 5 G
DIETARY FIBER: 1 G   SUGARS: 1 G   PROTEIN: 22 G

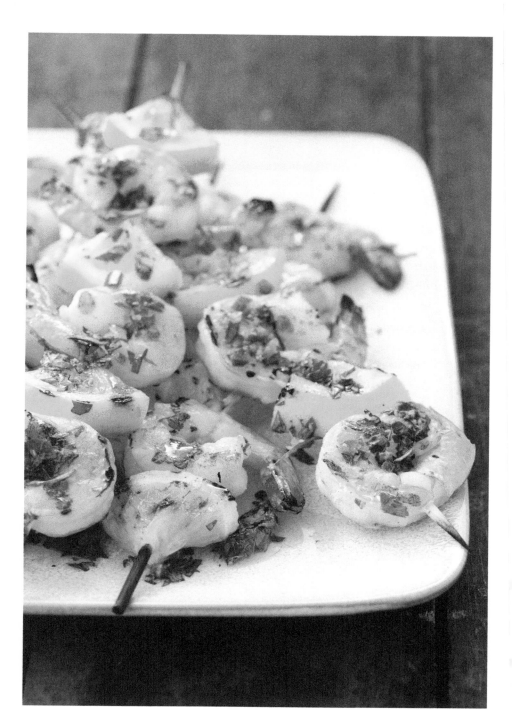

ROASTED SHRIMP
WITH TZATZIKI

Nut-Free

PREP TIME: 5 MINUTES ▲ COOK TIME: 10 MINUTES

SERVES 4   *Tzatziki is a garlicky, creamy sauce that is a staple in Greek cuisine. Here, roasted shrimp are tossed in this blend of Greek yogurt, chopped cucumbers, red onion, and of course, lots of garlic. Try serving with Roasted Beets with Yogurt (page 100) or Sautéed Dandelion Greens with Garlic (page 124).*

2 tablespoons regular olive oil

1 pound large shrimp, peeled and deveined

Sea salt

Freshly ground black pepper

¼ cup Tzatziki (page 278)

1 tablespoon chopped fresh oregano

1. Preheat the oven to 400°F.

2. In a baking dish, toss the shrimp with the oil, and season with salt and pepper. Roast in the oven for 8 to 10 minutes, or until opaque.

3. Transfer to a bowl, toss with the Tzatziki, and top with the oregano before serving.

PER SERVING   CALORIES: 176   FAT: 8 G   TOTAL CARBOHYDRATES: 5 G
DIETARY FIBER: 0 G   SUGARS: 1 G   PROTEIN: 23 G

THAI STEAMED MUSSELS WITH GINGER, LEMONGRASS, AND CHILES

Dairy-Free | Nut-Free | Paleo-Friendly

PREP TIME: 10 MINUTES ▲ COOK TIME: 10 MINUTES

SERVES 4   *With ginger, lemongrass, and chiles, the broth for these mussels takes on a distinctively Thai-inspired flair. Make sure to rinse them thoroughly under cold running water while scrubbing with a brush to remove any grit. Try serving these mussels over a bed of quinoa to soak up all the flavors.*

....

Ingredient Tip: Ask for farmed mussels at the seafood counter. They're already cleaned and rinsed, so you can get started cooking right away.

- 1 lemongrass stalk
- 2 pounds mussels, rinsed thoroughly and scrubbed
- 1 cup clam juice
- 1 cup vegetable broth
- 1 teaspoon fish sauce
- ½ cup chopped fresh ginger
- 2 serrano chiles, stemmed, seeded, and chopped

1. Remove and discard the tough outer layers of the lemongrass stalk, and thinly slice the tender core.

2. Place the mussels in a large pot. Add the lemongrass, clam juice, broth, fish sauce, ginger, and chiles.

3. Cover, bring to a boil, reduce to a simmer, and cook for about 5 minutes, or just until the mussels open. Discard any mussels that remain closed.

4. Ladle the mussels and the broth into bowls to serve.

PER SERVING   CALORIES: 274   FAT: 6 G   TOTAL CARBOHYDRATES: 23 G
DIETARY FIBER: 2 G   SUGARS: 3 G   PROTEIN: 30 G

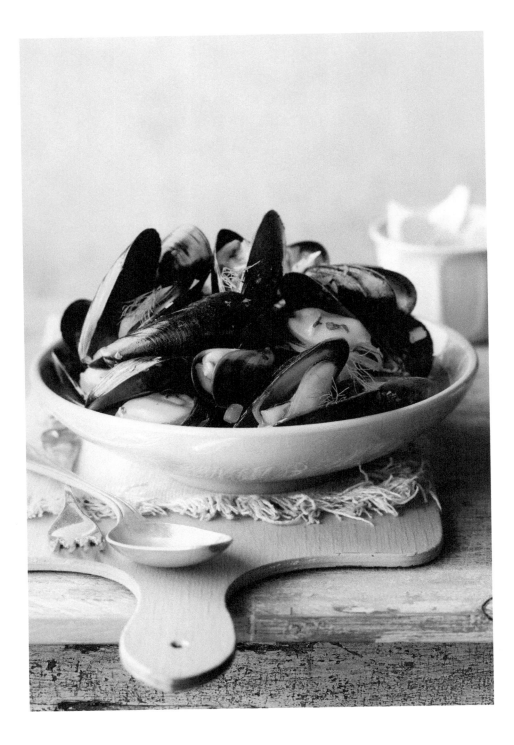

STEAMED MUSSELS WITH PARSLEY, LEMON, AND SHALLOT

Dairy-Free | Nut-Free | Paleo-Friendly

PREP TIME: 10 MINUTES ▲ COOK TIME: 10 MINUTES

SERVES 4   *Mussels, steamed in white wine and clam juice, are frequently found on bistro menus throughout the world. When choosing mussels at the store, make sure they are fresh and live—any open mussels should close when gently rapped on a counter. If they don't close, discard them.*

- **2 pounds mussels, rinsed thoroughly and scrubbed**
- **1 cup clam juice**
- **1 cup white wine**
- **½ cup chopped fresh flat-leaf parsley**
- **Juice of 1 lemon**
- **1 shallot, thinly sliced**
- **¼ cup torn dill sprigs, for garnish (optional)**

1. Place the mussels in a large pot.

2. Add the clam juice, white wine, parsley, lemon juice, and shallot. Cover, bring to a boil, reduce to a simmer, and cook for about 5 minutes, or just until the mussels open.

3. Transfer to bowls with the broth, and discard any mussels that remain closed. Garnish with the dill (if using).

PER SERVING CALORIES: 288 FAT: 5 G TOTAL CARBOHYDRATES: 20 G
DIETARY FIBER: 1 G SUGARS: 3 G PROTEIN: 28 G

PAN-SEARED TILAPIA WITH OLIVE TAPENADE AND LEMON ZEST

Dairy-Free | Nut-Free | Paleo-Friendly

PREP TIME: 5 MINUTES ▲ COOK TIME: 5 MINUTES

SERVES 4 *Because tilapia is a mild fish, it readily takes on the flavor of other ingredients. If you're looking for a side dish to go with this, try the Grilled Zucchini and Eggplant Salad with Feta and Red Onion (page 153).*

2 tablespoons regular olive oil

4 tilapia fillets

Sea salt

Freshly ground black pepper

3 tablespoons Olive Tapenade (page 284)

Zest of 1 lemon

2 tablespoons finely chopped fresh flat-leaf parsley

1. In a large skillet, heat the oil over high heat until it is almost smoking.

2. Pat the fillets dry, and season with salt and pepper. Add the tilapia fillets, and cook for 2 to 2½ minutes per side, or until golden brown. Using a fish spatula, remove the fillets from the pan, and transfer them to plates.

3. Serve the fish topped with the Olive Tapenade, lemon zest, and parsley.

PER SERVING CALORIES: 196 FAT: 12 G TOTAL CARBOHYDRATES: 1 G DIETARY FIBER: 1 G SUGARS: 0 G PROTEIN: 21 G

SHRIMP SCAMPI WITH QUINOA

Nut-Free

PREP TIME: 10 MINUTES ▲ COOK TIME: 15 MINUTES

SERVES 4   *Shrimp scampi is surprisingly easy to make. The combination of butter, garlic, lemon juice, fresh parsley, and shrimp is greater than the sum of its parts. The secret to its success lies in hitting all three major flavors of the dish and keeping them in balance: salt, fat, and acidity. Pair with a crisp glass of sauvignon blanc or pinot grigio.*

Diet Variation: To make this dairy-free, you can use olive oil instead of butter. If you want a rich flavor similar to butter, try equal amounts of coconut oil.

- **2 cups water**
- **1 cup quinoa**
- **¼ cup unsalted butter**
- **5 garlic cloves, thinly sliced**
- **1 pound large shrimp, peeled and deveined**
- **Sea salt**
- **Freshly ground black pepper**
- **Juice of 2 lemons**
- **½ cup finely chopped fresh parsley**

1. In a small pot, bring the water to a boil.
2. Add the quinoa, reduce the heat to a simmer, cover, and cook for about 12 minutes, or until all of the water is absorbed and the hard white center of each seed is no longer visible.
3. Meanwhile, in a large skillet, melt the butter over medium heat. Add the garlic, and cook for 1 minute, or until golden. »

4. Season the shrimp with salt and pepper, add to the skillet, and sauté for 1½ minutes per side, or just until they are opaque.

5. Turn off the heat, add the lemon juice and parsley, and serve the shrimp atop the quinoa.

PER SERVING CALORIES: 357 FAT: 14 G TOTAL CARBOHYDRATES: 32 G
DIETARY FIBER: 4 G SUGARS: 1 G PROTEIN: 28 G

PAN-FRIED TROUT WITH BLACK PEPPERCORN– BUTTERMILK DRESSING

PREP TIME: 5 MINUTES ▲ COOK TIME: 10 MINUTES

SERVES 4   *Deliciously crisp and quick to make, these pan-fried trout fillets are a great option for busy weeknights. Almond meal is used in place of flour. Every bite is accompanied with a tangy, creamy, and pleasantly peppery buttermilk dressing that comes together in just minutes. The peppercorns are added to the buttermilk dressing as a spicy contrast to its richness. Serve with Southern-Style Collard Greens with Smoked Bacon (page 130) or Honey-Roasted Carrots (page 133).*

Cooking Tip: When placing fish fillets into a hot pan, allow one end of the fillet to touch the side of the pan closest to you, and gently let the other side drop into the oil away from your body.

    ¼ cup almond meal
    Sea salt
    4 rainbow trout fillets
    1 egg, beaten
    ¼ cup regular olive oil
    3 tablespoons Buttermilk Dressing (page 289)
    10 whole black peppercorns, crushed

1. Place the almond meal on a plate, and season with salt generously. Pat the trout fillets dry, and dredge them in the egg followed by the almond meal. Shake off any excess. »

2. In a large skillet, heat the oil over medium-high heat. Add the fillets, and cook for 3 to 4 minutes per side, or until golden. Using a fish spatula, carefully remove the fillets and drain on paper towels.

3. In a small bowl, mix together the Buttermilk Dressing and peppercorns. Transfer the fillets to plates, and top with the dressing before serving.

PER SERVING CALORIES: 363 FAT: 29 G TOTAL CARBOHYDRATES: 2 G
DIETARY FIBER: 1 G SUGARS: 0 G PROTEIN: 25 G

BAKED TILAPIA WITH GINGER AND SCALLIONS

Dairy-Free | Nut-Free | Paleo-Friendly

PREP TIME: 5 MINUTES ▲ COOK TIME: 15 MINUTES

SERVES 4   *The tilapia fillets stay moist as they bake in an Asian-inspired mixture of fish sauce, toasted sesame oil, fresh grated ginger, and chopped scallions. Sautéed Spinach with Nutmeg (page 119) or Roasted Asparagus with Garlic and Orange Zest (page 128) make great sides.*

1 tablespoon toasted sesame oil

1 tablespoon fish sauce

¼ cup vegetable broth

1 tablespoon grated fresh ginger

¼ cup chopped scallions, white and green parts

4 tilapia fillets

1. Preheat the oven to 425°F.

2. In a small bowl, mix together the sesame oil, fish sauce, broth, ginger, and scallions.

3. Place the fish fillets in an ovenproof skillet with a lid, just large enough to fit them all snugly.

4. Pour the mixture over the fish fillets, cover with the lid, and bake in the oven for 10 to 15 minutes, or until the fillets are cooked through.

PER SERVING   CALORIES: 134   FAT: 5 G   TOTAL CARBOHYDRATES: 2 G
DIETARY FIBER: 0 G   SUGARS: 0 G   PROTEIN: 22 G

SEARED CALAMARI WITH LEMON AND CAPERS

Dairy-Free | Nut-Free | Paleo-Friendly

PREP TIME: 5 MINUTES ▲ COOK TIME: 5 MINUTES

SERVES 4   *These days, calamari is in vogue. Why? Because it's a sustainable source of seafood and it's delicious and cooks quickly. Most people are familiar with calamari from Italian American restaurants, where it is often breaded, fried, and served with marinara sauce as an appetizer. But you can get a lot more creative with calamari than that—and make something healthier as well. Here it is quickly sautéed to render it pleasantly crisp around the edges without turning the center rubbery, and its rich flavor pairs nicely with the acidity of capers and lemon.*

1 tablespoon regular olive oil

1 pound whole calamari bodies with tentacles, cleaned

Sea salt

Freshly ground black pepper

Juice of ½ lemon

1 tablespoon capers

2 tablespoons finely chopped fresh flat-leaf parsley

5 cherry tomatoes, chopped, for garnish (optional)

Zest of ½ lemon, for garnish (optional)

½ cup torn basil leaves, for garnish (optional)

1. In a large skillet, heat the oil over high heat until it is almost smoking.

2. Season the calamari with salt and pepper, add to the pan, and sear for 2 to 3 minutes, or just until cooked through.

3. Add the lemon juice, capers, and parsley, heat through for 15 seconds, and transfer to serving plates. Garnish with the tomatoes, lemon zest, and basil (if using).

PER SERVING   CALORIES: 140   FAT: 8 G   TOTAL CARBOHYDRATES: 9 G
DIETARY FIBER: 1 G   SUGARS: 0 G   PROTEIN: 8 G

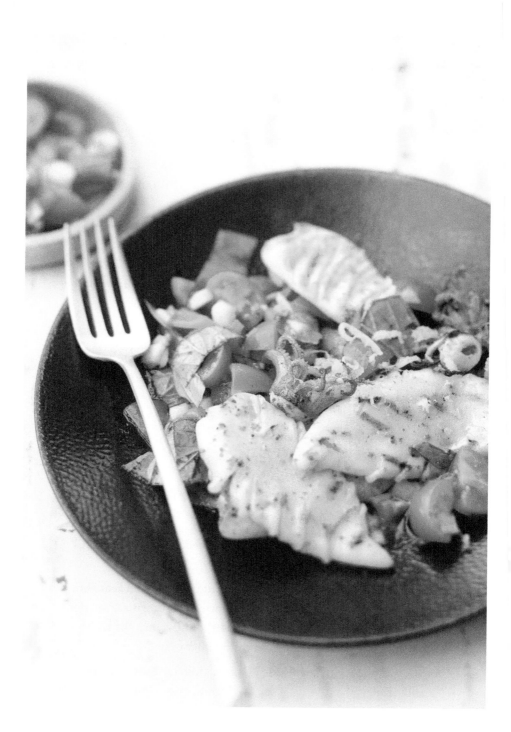

PAN-ROASTED SALMON WITH PICKLED ONIONS AND MUSTARD VINAIGRETTE

Dairy-Free | Nut-Free | Paleo-Friendly

PREP TIME: 5 MINUTES ⌄ COOK TIME: 10 MINUTES

SERVES 4   *Whenever possible, choose wild Alaskan salmon (even when frozen) over farmed salmon for its superior omega-3 fatty acid content, responsible environmental stewardship, and most importantly, better flavor. Pair with a classic side such as Roasted Asparagus with Garlic and Orange Zest (page 128).*

Ingredient Tip: Wild Alaskan salmon is a seasonal product. Look for fresh fillets during the summer and frozen fillets during other times of the year.

- 2 tablespoons regular olive oil
- 1 pound salmon fillets
- Sea salt
- Freshly ground black pepper
- ¼ cup Pickled Onions (page 291)
- 3 tablespoons Mustard Vinaigrette (page 287)
- 2 tablespoons finely chopped fresh flat-leaf parsley

1. Preheat the oven to 350°F.

2. Heat the oil in an ovenproof pan over medium-high heat until almost smoking.

3. Pat the salmon dry, season with salt and pepper, and sear skin side down for about 5 minutes, or until a crust forms. Transfer to the oven, and roast for 5 to 7 minutes, or just until the tip of a paring knife pierces the center of the fillet easily.

4. Serve topped with the Pickled Onions, Mustard Vinaigrette, and parsley.

PER SERVING   CALORIES: 307   FAT: 21 G   TOTAL CARBOHYDRATES: 6 G
DIETARY FIBER: 1 G   SUGARS: 4 G   PROTEIN: 23 G

GRILLED BRANZINO WITH EASY PICO DE GALLO

Dairy-Free | Nut-Free | Paleo-Friendly

PREP TIME: 5 MINUTES ▲ COOK TIME: 10 MINUTES

SERVES 4 *Branzino is a Mediterranean fish that doesn't need much in the way of preparation. The simpler, the better. Here, it's grilled whole on the bone and served with pico de gallo, a mixture of chopped tomatoes, onions, and jalapeño pepper. If you can't find whole branzino, striped bass or bluefish fillets are good substitutes. Serve with a grilled side such as Mexican Grilled Corn (page 117).*

Ingredient Tip: Branzino also sometimes goes by the name Mediterranean sea bass.

2 whole branzinos, about 1 pound each

2 tablespoons regular olive oil

Sea salt

Freshly ground black pepper

¼ cup Easy Pico de Gallo (page 270)

1. Prepare a gas or charcoal grill for medium-high-heat cooking.

2. Pat the fish dry, coat with oil, and season with salt and pepper.

3. Grill the fish for about 5 minutes per side, or until the skin is crisp and the flesh is easily pierced with a fork and juicy.

4. To remove the fillets from the fish, lay the fish on its side, and insert the tip of the knife near the head along the top of the spine. Gently cut along the spine toward the tail, and lift the top fillet off using the flat side of the knife. Using your hands, lift the bone away from the bottom fillet—it should come off easily in one piece. Serve topped with the Easy Pico de Gallo.

PER SERVING   CALORIES: 309   FAT: 13 G   TOTAL CARBOHYDRATES: 1 G
DIETARY FIBER: 0 G   SUGARS: 0 G   PROTEIN: 47 G

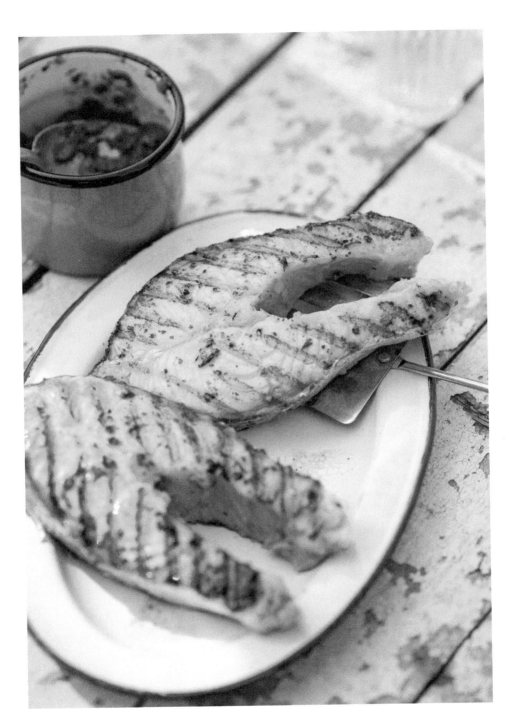

GRILLED SALMON WITH OLIVE TAPENADE

Dairy-Free | Nut-Free | Paleo-Friendly

PREP TIME: 5 MINUTES ⨯ COOK TIME: 10 MINUTES

SERVES 4   *When grilling fish, resist the urge to move it around on the grill. If you keep moving the fish around, you won't get those coveted grill marks. Even firm-fleshed fish must be handled minimally to keep their flesh from falling apart as it cooks. Pair this dish with a full-bodied white wine such as a California chardonnay or a light-bodied red wine such as pinot noir.*

1 pound salmon fillets, cut into 4-ounce pieces

2 tablespoons regular olive oil

Sea salt

Freshly ground black pepper

3 tablespoons Olive Tapenade (page 284)

1. Prepare a gas or charcoal grill for high-heat cooking.

2. Pat the salmon dry, coat with the oil, and season with salt and pepper.

3. Grill the salmon with the lid closed for 3 to 4 minutes per side, or until the skin is crisp and the flesh is easily pierced with a fork.

4. Serve topped with the Olive Tapenade.

PER SERVING   CALORIES: 285   FAT: 22 G   TOTAL CARBOHYDRATES: 0 G
DIETARY FIBER: 0 G   SUGARS: 0 G   PROTEIN: 23 G

POACHED FRESH COD WITH GRAPE TOMATOES, CAPERS, AND OLIVES

Dairy-Free | Nut-Free | Paleo-Friendly

PREP TIME: 5 MINUTES ▲ COOK TIME: 16 MINUTES

SERVES 4   *Use the freshest cod you can find, preferably fillets that are similar in size and from the center of the fish. Poaching the fish takes less than 10 minutes, and when it's done, the delicious broth—a citrusy mixture of fine Mediterranean ingredients—doubles as a pan sauce.*

1 tablespoon extra-virgin olive oil

1 cup grape tomatoes, halved

3 garlic cloves, thinly sliced

2 tablespoons capers

1 tablespoon red pepper flakes

2 tablespoons chopped, pitted Kalamata olives

1 pound cod fillets, cut into 4-ounce portions

Sea salt

Freshly ground black pepper

½ cup white wine

½ cup vegetable broth

1. In a medium skillet, heat the oil over medium heat.

2. Add the tomatoes, garlic, capers, red pepper flakes, and olives, and cook for 3 to 5 minutes, or until the tomatoes have softened slightly and the garlic is golden.

3. Season both sides of the fish with salt and pepper, nestle the fish in the mixture, and add the white wine and broth (which should come about halfway up the fillets).

4. Bring the liquid to a gentle simmer, and poach for about 4 to 5 minutes, or until the fish is opaque on the sides. Using a fish spatula, carefully flip each fillet, using your free hand to hold the fish steady on the spatula. Cook the other side for about 4 to 5 minutes, or until the fish flakes easily in the center with a fork.

5. Serve the fish in shallow bowls with the broth.

PER SERVING CALORIES: 170 FAT: 6 G TOTAL CARBOHYDRATES: 4 G
DIETARY FIBER: 1 G SUGARS: 2 G PROTEIN: 22 G

CIOPPINO

Dairy-Free I Nut-Free I Paleo-Friendly

PREP TIME: 15 MINUTES ▲ COOK TIME: 20 MINUTES

SERVES 6   *Cioppino is a fisherman's stew that originated in San Francisco, with roots from the region of Liguria in northern Italy. It often incorporates the day's catch, simmering the fish and shellfish together in a tomato-based broth. Since the cooking time of each component is different, the seafood— in this case, mussels, shrimp, and black bass—is cooked separately and then simmered together at the end.*

> 2 tablespoons extra-virgin olive oil
>
> 1 tablespoon tomato paste
>
> 3 garlic cloves, thinly sliced
>
> ½ pound large shrimp
>
> Sea salt
>
> Freshly ground black pepper
>
> 1 cup clam juice
>
> 1 cup white wine
>
> ¼ cup finely chopped fresh flat-leaf parsley
>
> 1 pound mussels, rinsed thoroughly and scrubbed
>
> 1 (28-ounce) can whole peeled tomatoes
>
> ½ pound black bass fillets, cut into 1-inch pieces

1. In a large pot, heat the oil over medium heat.

2. Add the tomato paste and garlic, and cook for 1 minute, or until the garlic is golden.

3. Season the shrimp with salt and pepper, add to the pot, and cook for 1½ minutes per side, or just until opaque. Remove with a slotted spoon to a plate or cutting board. To the pot, add the clam juice, white wine, parsley, and mussels. Cover, bring to a boil, reduce to a simmer, and cook for about 5 minutes, or just until the mussels open. »

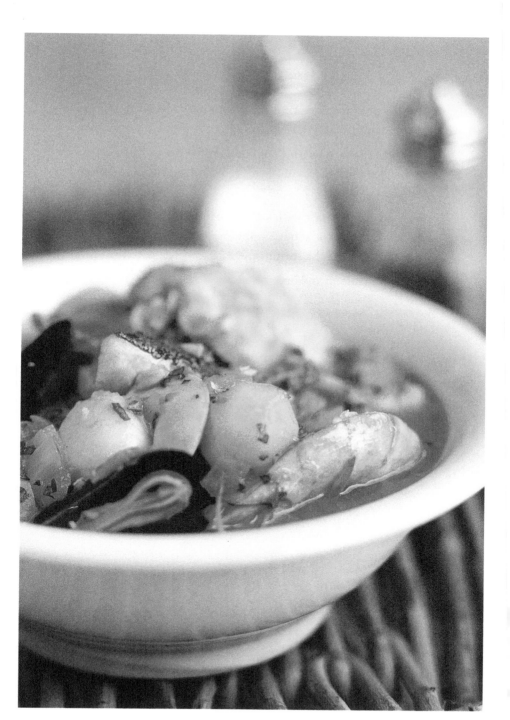

4. Using a slotted spoon, transfer the mussels to a bowl. Discard any that remain closed.

5. Place the tomatoes with their liquid in the bowl of a food processor, and process until smooth. Then add the tomatoes to the pot.

6. Season the black bass with salt and pepper, add the black bass to the pot, simmer for about 5 minutes, or just until cooked through, and add the shrimp and mussels back in to heat through.

7. Ladle the seafood and broth among 6 bowls.

PER SERVING   CALORIES: 251   FAT: 8 G   TOTAL CARBOHYDRATES: 15 G
DIETARY FIBER: 2 G   SUGARS: 6 G   PROTEIN: 25 G

SOUTH INDIAN–STYLE FISH CURRY

Nut-Free | Paleo-Friendly

PREP TIME: 5 MINUTES ▲ COOK TIME: 15 MINUTES

SERVES 4   *Mangalore is a coastal region in the southwest part of India, where seafood figures prominently into the regional cuisine. In this dish, inspired by a Mangalorean style of preparing fish curry, tender pieces of fish are simmered in a mixture of coconut milk, vinegar, turmeric, and chiles. The curry leans toward the hot side, so if you're heat shy, use fewer chiles. Pair with a semisweet, fruity white wine such as a white burgundy or a kabinett riesling, which will help offset the heat and acidity of the dish.*

1 tablespoon unsalted butter

½ red onion, sliced

1 pound tilapia fillets, cut into 1-inch pieces

1 teaspoon ground turmeric

Sea salt

Freshly ground black pepper

1 (15-ounce) can coconut milk

2 tablespoons distilled white vinegar

5 sprigs cilantro

2 serrano chiles, stemmed, seeded, and chopped

Juice of 1 lime

1. In a medium pot, melt the butter over medium heat.

2. Add the onion, and cook for 5 to 7 minutes, or until crisp-tender.

3. Season the tilapia fillets with the turmeric, salt, and pepper, and add to the pot. Add the coconut milk, vinegar, cilantro, »

and chiles, and bring to a simmer. Cook for about 5 minutes, or just until the fish is easily flaked with a fork.

4. Remove from the heat, and stir in the lime juice. Divide the fish and broth among four bowls.

PER SERVING   CALORIES: 380   FAT: 29 G   TOTAL CARBOHYDRATES: 10 G
DIETARY FIBER: 3 G   SUGARS: 5 G   PROTEIN: 24 G

SEARED SCALLOPS WITH PICKLED ONIONS AND CHARMOULA

Dairy-Free | Nut-Free | Paleo-Friendly

PREP TIME: 5 MINUTES ▲ COOK TIME: 5 MINUTES

SERVES 4 *For an interesting twist, add some chopped chiles to the pickled onions to turn them into a spicy relish. Or season them with a pinch of cayenne pepper just before placing them atop the scallops. Accompany with a side of quinoa and a refreshing salad like Arugula Salad with Radishes, Pomegranate Seeds, and Pine Nuts (page 139) for a satisfying and delicious meal.*

Cooking Tip: Make sure to pat the scallops dry before adding them to the pan, or they won't brown properly.

>   2 tablespoons regular olive oil
>   1 pound dry-packed sea scallops
>   Sea salt
>   Freshly ground black pepper
>   2 tablespoons Charmoula (page 283)
>   ¼ cup Pickled Onions (page 291)

1. In a large skillet, heat the oil over high heat until almost smoking.

2. Season the scallops with salt and pepper. Place the scallops in a single layer in the pan, and cook, undisturbed, for 1½ minutes, or until a brown crust forms. Using a pair of tongs, gently turn the scallops, and cook for 1½ minutes, or just before they are cooked through. (If the scallops do not release easily, allow them to cook longer, and shake the pan to loosen.)

3. Using tongs, transfer the scallops to plates, drizzle with the Charmoula, and top with the Pickled Onions.

PER SERVING CALORIES: 214 FAT: 12 G TOTAL CARBOHYDRATES: 6 G
DIETARY FIBER: 0 G SUGARS: 2 G PROTEIN: 19 G

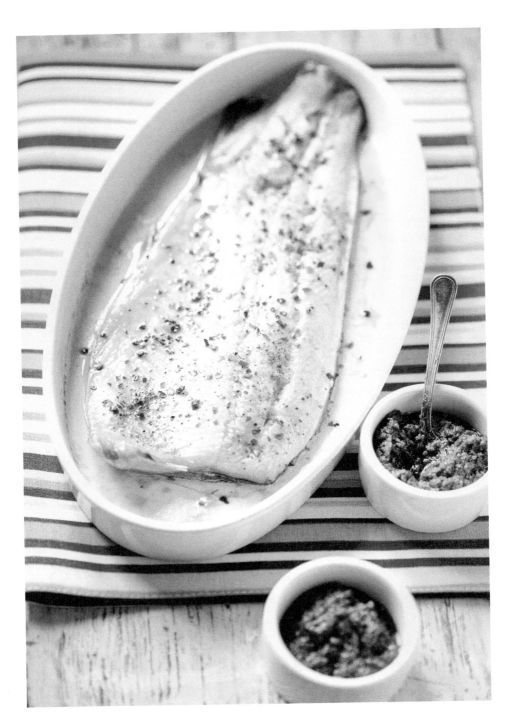

PAN-ROASTED TROUT
WITH PESTO

Dairy-Free | Nut-Free | Paleo-Friendly

PREP TIME: 5 MINUTES ▲ COOK TIME: 15 MINUTES

SERVES 4　*Farmed rainbow trout from the United States is one of the few sustainably raised sources of farmed fish and was recently named a best choice by the Monterey Bay Aquarium's Seafood Watch. Serve this quick-cooking main with a side of leafy greens, like Sautéed Dandelion Greens with Garlic (page 124), or some Snappy Green Beans with Lemon Zest and Olive Tapenade (page 120).*

2 tablespoons regular olive oil

4 rainbow trout fillets

Sea salt

Freshly ground black pepper

3 tablespoons Simple Basil Pesto (page 274)

1. Preheat the oven to 400°F.

2. In a large, ovenproof skillet, heat the oil over high heat until it is almost smoking.

3. Pat the fish dry on both sides gently with a kitchen towel. Season the fish with salt and pepper.

4. Place the fish fillets skin side down in the oil, and cook for about 1 minute, or until a golden crust forms. Transfer to the oven, and roast for about 10 to 12 minutes, or just until cooked through.

5. Serve the fish with the Simple Basil Pesto on top.

PER SERVING　CALORIES: 261　FAT: 19 G　TOTAL CARBOHYDRATES: 0 G
DIETARY FIBER: 0 G　SUGARS: 0 G　PROTEIN: 23 G

SHRIMP FRA DIAVOLO

Dairy-Free | Nut-Free | Paleo-Friendly

PREP TIME: 5 MINUTES ▲ COOK TIME: 10 MINUTES

SERVES 4   *This Italian American classic has a bit of a devilish side to it. In fact, the name means "brother devil" when translated. And it's easy to see why: The shrimp is simmered in a spicy tomato sauce that packs some serious heat from red pepper flakes. This recipe uses a jalapeño pepper for even more heat, but feel free to leave it out.*

Ingredient Tip: As a rule of thumb, the smaller the hot pepper, the hotter it will be. For example, the mighty habañero pepper is tiny in size compared to, say, a jalapeño pepper, but it packs an outsized dose of heat.

- 2 tablespoons regular olive oil
- 3 garlic cloves, chopped
- 3 tablespoons red pepper flakes
- 1 jalapeño pepper, stemmed, seeded, and chopped
- 1 pound large shrimp, peeled and deveined
- Sea salt
- Freshly ground black pepper
- 1 cup Quick Marinara Sauce (page 272)
- ¼ cup white wine

1. In a large skillet, heat the oil over medium heat.

2. Add the garlic, red pepper flakes, and jalapeño, and cook for 1 minute, or until the garlic is golden.

3. Season the shrimp with salt and pepper, add to the skillet, and cook for 1 minute.

196   LOSE WHEAT IN 4 WEEKS

4. Add the Quick Marinara Sauce and wine, bring to a simmer, and cook for 2 minutes, or just until the shrimp is opaque.

5. Divide the shrimp among 4 plates, and serve topped with the sauce.

PER SERVING   CALORIES: 234   FAT: 11 G   TOTAL CARBOHYDRATES: 11 G
DIETARY FIBER: 3 G   SUGARS: 4 G   PROTEIN: 23 G

CHAPTER 10

Meat and Poultry

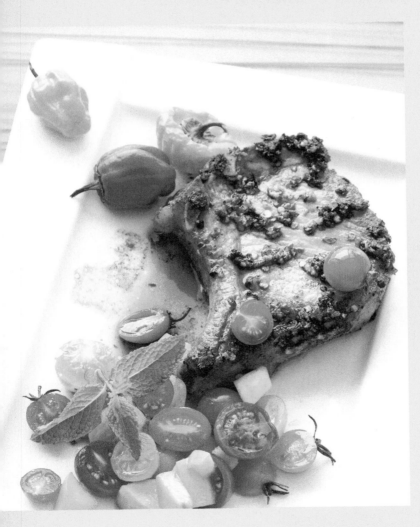

SHISH KABOBS WITH CHIMICHURRI

Dairy-Free | Nut-Free | Paleo-Friendly

PREP TIME: 10 MINUTES ▲ COOK TIME: 10 MINUTES

SERVES 4   *Shish kabobs are traditionally Middle Eastern skewers of lamb cooked over an open fire. In this recipe steak is used, but lamb or chicken works just as well. Finish with tangy chimichurri sauce.*

- 1 pound sirloin steak, cut into 1-inch cubes
- 1 red onion, roughly chopped
- 1 green bell pepper, roughly chopped
- 1 beefsteak tomato, roughly chopped
- 2 tablespoons regular olive oil
- Sea salt
- Freshly ground black pepper
- ¼ cup Chimichurri (page 282)

1. If using wooden skewers, soak 12 skewers in water for 15 minutes. Prepare a gas or charcoal grill for high-heat cooking.

2. In a large mixing bowl, toss the steak, onion, bell pepper, and tomato in the oil, and season with salt and pepper. Thread onto the skewers, alternating pieces of steak with the vegetables.

3. Grill for 2 to 3 minutes per side, or until the steak reads 130°F for medium rare on an instant-read thermometer.

4. Put 3 skewers per plate on 4 plates. Serve with the Chimichurri drizzled on top.

PER SERVING   CALORIES: 398   FAT: 26 G   TOTAL CARBOHYDRATES: 6 G
DIETARY FIBER: 2 G   SUGARS: 3 G   PROTEIN: 35 G

PAN-ROASTED PORK CHOPS WITH CHERRY TOMATOES

Dairy-Free | Nut-Free | Paleo-Friendly

PREP TIME: 5 MINUTES ▲ COOK TIME: 15 MINUTES

SERVES 4   *These pork chops, seared on the stovetop to achieve a golden-brown crust and finished in the oven just until cooked through, are served with cherry tomatoes. Pair with a light-bodied, citrusy wine such as a young sauvignon blanc or verdejo.*

2 tablespoons regular olive oil

4 bone-in pork chops

Sea salt

Freshly ground black pepper

1 cup cherry tomatoes, halved

1. Preheat the oven to 375°F.

2. In a large, ovenproof skillet, heat the oil over high heat until almost smoking.

3. Season the pork chops with salt and pepper. Add the pork chops to the skillet, and cook for about 3 minutes, or until browned on one side. Flip the pork chops, and transfer the skillet to the oven. Roast for about 10 minutes, or until an instant-read thermometer inserted into the center of the chops reads 145°F.

4. Divide the chops among plates and serve with the cherry tomatoes.

PER SERVING CALORIES: 323 FAT: 20 G TOTAL CARBOHYDRATES: 1 G
DIETARY FIBER: 0 G SUGARS: 0 G PROTEIN: 30 G

CITRUS-MARINATED GRILLED SKIRT STEAK SALAD

Dairy-Free | Nut-Free | Paleo-Friendly

PREP TIME: 5 MINUTES (PLUS MARINATING TIME) ▲ COOK TIME: 10 MINUTES

SERVES 4 *Looking for a salad that's substantial enough to serve as a hearty meal? Here's one that's definitely worth trying. The juicy, marinated, perfectly grilled steak will ensure this recipe makes it into the weekly lunch rotation. You'll probably have more steak than you need, so save any extra for another preparation like Grilled Skirt Steak with Chimichurri (page 210).*

Cooking Tip: Cuts like skirt steak and flank steak are best cooked to medium-rare since they tend to become chewy the longer they are cooked. They should also be sliced against the grain for the same reason.

- **2¼ pounds skirt steak**
- **¼ cup regular olive oil**
- **Juice of 3 lemons**
- **Sea salt**
- **Freshly ground black pepper**
- **1 bunch arugula**
- **1 pint cherry tomatoes, halved**
- **½ red onion, sliced**
- **3 tablespoons Mustard Vinaigrette (page 287), divided**

1. Place the steak, oil, and lemon juice in a zipper-close bag and marinate for 10 to 15 minutes.

2. Meanwhile, prepare a gas or charcoal grill for high-heat cooking.

3. Season the skirt steak with salt and pepper. Grill the steak for about 4 minutes per side, or until an instant-read thermometer reads 130°F for medium rare.

4. Let the steak rest for at least 10 minutes before slicing against the grain. In a large bowl, toss together the arugula, cherry tomatoes, onion, and 2 tablespoons of Mustard Vinaigrette.

5. Divide the salad among 4 plates, and top each with the steak. Drizzle the remaining 1 tablespoon of Mustard Vinaigrette over the steak.

PER SERVING   CALORIES: 739   FAT: 46 G   TOTAL CARBOHYDRATES: 10 G
DIETARY FIBER: 3 G   SUGARS: 4 G   PROTEIN: 71 G

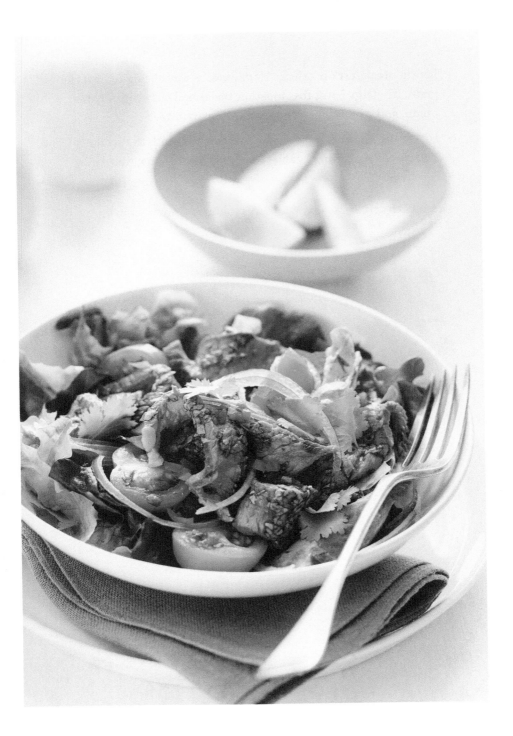

SPICY THAI BEEF SALAD

Dairy-Free | Nut-Free | Paleo-Friendly

PREP TIME: 10 MINUTES ▲ COOK TIME: 10 MINUTES

SERVES 6   *Each bite of* Yum Nuea, *or northeastern Thai beef salad, has a bit of charred smokiness from the grilled meat, richness from the fish sauce, tartness from the lime, and of course, heat from the chiles. It's quick to prepare, making it a great option for a casual lunch. Serve with a fruity white wine to balance the acidity and heat.*

> 1 lemongrass stalk
>
> 3 tablespoons toasted sesame oil
>
> Juice of 1 lime
>
> 1 teaspoon fish sauce
>
> 2 serrano chile peppers, stemmed, seeded, and finely chopped
>
> 2¼ pounds skirt steak
>
> 2 tablespoons regular olive oil
>
> Sea salt
>
> Freshly ground white pepper
>
> ½ head lettuce, chopped
>
> ½ red onion, thinly sliced
>
> 1 beefsteak tomato, chopped

1. Remove and discard the tough outer layers of the lemongrass stalk, and thinly slice the tender core.

2. In a medium bowl, whisk the sesame oil into the lime juice and fish sauce. Add the chiles and lemongrass, and set aside.

3. Prepare a gas or charcoal grill for high-heat cooking. »

4. Coat the steak with the olive oil, and season with salt and pepper. Grill the steak for 4 minutes per side, or until an instant-read thermometer reads 130°F for medium rare.

5. Let the meat rest for 10 minutes before slicing against the grain. In a bowl, toss the sliced steak with the lettuce, onion, tomato, and sesame oil dressing.

PER SERVING CALORIES: 466 FAT: 29 G TOTAL CARBOHYDRATES: 4 G
DIETARY FIBER: 1 G SUGARS: 2 G PROTEIN: 46 G

THAI STIR-FRIED BEEF

Dairy-Free

PREP TIME: 15 MINUTES ▲ COOK TIME: 8 MINUTES

SERVES 4   *Sweet, sour, spicy, and salty—this easy stir-fry has it all. The hallmark of just about any dish in Thai cooking is to have each of these elements in balance. This stir-fry is also a nutritious meal, with plenty of crisp-tender vegetables to go with the beef. If you like, you can try this dish with pork tenderloin.*

Cooking Tip: With any stir-fry recipe, measure and prep all of the ingredients before you start because stir-frying requires constant cooking and you won't have time to stop.

- **1 pound sirloin steak**
- **3 teaspoons regular olive oil, divided**
- **3 garlic cloves, chopped**
- **1 serrano chile, stemmed, seeded, and chopped**
- **½ bunch asparagus, trimmed and cut into bite-size pieces**
- **1 pound spinach, stemmed**
- **1 teaspoon fish sauce**
- **¼ cup Homemade Peanut Sauce (page 292)**
- **Juice of 1 lime**

1. To make the steak easier to slice, place in the freezer for about 10 to 15 minutes, then slice about ⅛-inch thick against the grain.

2. In a wok or large skillet, heat 1 teaspoon of oil over high heat until almost smoking. Add the garlic and chile, and cook for about 10 seconds, stirring constantly.

3. Add the steak, and cook for about 2 to 3 minutes, stirring constantly, or until slightly pink in the center. Remove with a slotted spoon to a bowl. »

4. Heat the remaining 2 teaspoons of olive oil over high heat until it is almost smoking. Add the asparagus, and cook for 2 to 3 minutes, stirring constantly, or until crisp-tender. Add the spinach, and cook for 1 minute, stirring constantly, or until just wilted.

5. Add the fish sauce and Peanut Sauce, cook for 1 minute, stirring, or until heated through, and add the lime juice and steak.

6. Divide among 4 plates, and serve immediately.

PER SERVING   CALORIES: 353   FAT: 16 G   TOTAL CARBOHYDRATES: 14 G
DIETARY FIBER: 6 G   SUGARS: 5 G   PROTEIN: 42 G

GRILLED PORK CHOPS WITH ONIONS AND BUTTERMILK DRESSING

Nut-Free

PREP TIME: 10 MINUTES ▲ COOK TIME: 10 MINUTES

SERVES 4   *Bone-in pork chops turn tender and juicy on a hot grill. The Buttermilk Dressing adds a tangy flavor and the Pickled Onions bring in a sweet-tart taste. The toppings are easily prepared while the grill is preheating. Mexican Grilled Corn (page 117) and Greek Yogurt Potato Salad with Fresh Herbs (page 98) are great accompaniments. Serve with your favorite glass of white wine.*

   4 bone-in pork chops
   2 tablespoons regular olive oil
   Sea salt
   Freshly ground black pepper
   ½ cup Pickled Onions (page 291)
   ¼ cup Buttermilk Dressing (page 289)

1. Prepare a gas or charcoal grill for medium-heat cooking.

2. Coat the pork chops with oil, and season with salt and pepper. Grill the chops for 3 to 4 minutes per side, or until grill marks appear and an instant-read thermometer inserted into the center without touching the bone reads 145°F.

3. Serve with the Pickled Onions and Buttermilk Dressing on top.

PER SERVING   CALORIES: 399   FAT: 36 G   TOTAL CARBOHYDRATES: 0 G
DIETARY FIBER: 0 G   SUGARS: 0 G   PROTEIN: 18 G

GRILLED SKIRT STEAK
WITH CHIMICHURRI

Dairy-Free | Nut-Free | Paleo-Friendly

PREP TIME: 5 MINUTES ▲ COOK TIME: 10 MINUTES

SERVES 8   *Chimichurri, an Argentinean condiment that's often served with grilled meats, is a snap to prepare. It's made with parsley, cilantro, garlic, red wine vinegar, and extra-virgin olive oil. Since chimichurri packs a punch, a little goes a long way.*

Cooking Tip: Always bring meats to room temperature before grilling to ensure even cooking.

2¼ pounds skirt steak

2 tablespoons extra-virgin olive oil

Sea salt

Freshly ground black pepper

½ cup Chimichurri (page 282)

1. Prepare a gas or charcoal grill for high-heat cooking.

2. Coat the skirt steak with the oil, and season with salt and pepper.

3. Grill the steak for about 4 minutes per side, or until an instant-read thermometer reads 130°F for medium rare.

4. Let the meat rest for at least 10 minutes before slicing against the grain. Top with the Chimichurri before serving.

PER SERVING CALORIES: 370 FAT: 25 G TOTAL CARBOHYDRATES: 1 G
DIETARY FIBER: 1 G SUGARS: 0 G PROTEIN: 34 G

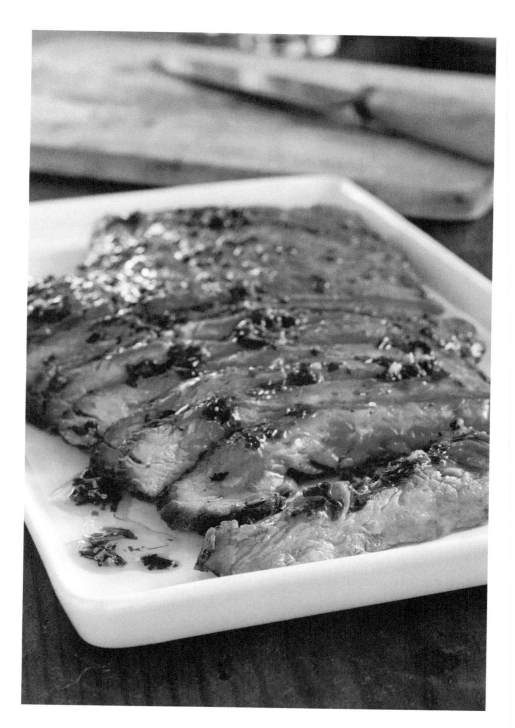

PAN-ROASTED PORK CHOPS WITH BEAN SPROUTS AND PEAS

Dairy-Free | Nut-Free

PREP TIME: 5 MINUTES ⬥ COOK TIME: 10 MINUTES

SERVES 4   *In the spring, when fresh peas are in season, this easy dish will help you make the transition away from comfort food toward lighter fare.*

2 tablespoons regular olive oil

4 (4-ounce) boneless pork chops

Sea salt

Freshly ground black pepper

½ cup shelled English peas

½ cup sugar snap peas

1 cup bean sprouts

½ cup mixed greens

1. Preheat the oven to 375°F.

2. In a large, ovenproof skillet, heat the oil over high heat until almost smoking.

3. Season the pork chops with salt and pepper. Add the pork chops to the skillet, and cook for about 3 minutes, or until browned on one side. Flip the pork chops, and transfer the skillet to the oven. Roast for about 5 to 7 minutes, or until an instant-read thermometer inserted into the center of the chops reads 145°F.

4. Meanwhile, bring a medium pot of water to a boil over high heat, and fill a medium bowl with ice water.

5. Blanch the peas for 3 to 4 minutes, or until bright green and tender.

6. Transfer the peas to the ice water. Drain well.

7. Divide the chops among 4 plates. Serve with the peas, bean sprouts, and mixed greens, and drizzle with the pan juices.

PER SERVING   CALORIES: 274   FAT: 11 G   TOTAL CARBOHYDRATES: 9 G
DIETARY FIBER: 2 G   SUGARS: 2 G   PROTEIN: 34 G

PORK CHOPS ALLA PIZZAIOLA

Dairy-Free | Nut-Free | Paleo-Friendly

PREP TIME: 5 MINUTES ▲ COOK TIME: 20 MINUTES

SERVES 4 *Here's something that kids and adults will probably be able to agree on at the dinner table: pork chops simmered in pizza sauce. They're delicious. It's amazing what you can do just by adding a couple of key ingredients to a base sauce. Bone-in pork chops are preferred because they're juicier, but you can use boneless if you prefer.*

> 2 tablespoons regular olive oil
>
> 4 bone-in pork chops
>
> Sea salt
>
> Freshly ground black pepper
>
> 3 garlic cloves, chopped
>
> 1 tablespoon red pepper flakes
>
> 1 teaspoon dried oregano
>
> 2 cups Quick Marinara Sauce (page 272)

1. Preheat the oven to 375°F.

2. In a large, ovenproof skillet with a lid, heat the oil over high heat until it is almost smoking.

3. Season the pork chops with salt and pepper, and cook for about 3 minutes, or until browned on one side. Remove the pork chops to a plate, and reduce the heat to medium.

4. Add the garlic, red pepper flakes, and oregano to the skillet and cook for 1 minute. Add the Quick Marinara Sauce and bring to a simmer. Return the pork chops to the skillet, cover with a lid, and transfer to the oven for about 10 minutes, or until an instant-read thermometer inserted into the center reads 145°F.

5. Transfer the pork chops to 4 plates, and serve topped with the sauce.

PER SERVING   CALORIES: 433   FAT: 34 G   TOTAL CARBOHYDRATES: 13 G
DIETARY FIBER: 5 G   SUGARS: 7 G   PROTEIN: 21 G

PROVENÇAL-STYLE LAMB STEW

Dairy-Free | Nut-Free

PREP TIME: 10 MINUTES ⌄ COOK TIME: 35 MINUTES

SERVES 8   *Lamb shoulder is a particularly good cut for stewing since it turns tender with slow cooking. Serve with a piping hot cup of Mulled Wine with Cinnamon, Citrus, and Clove (page 267) for the ultimate cold weather indulgence.*

Diet Variation: To cut down on the amount of carbohydrates in this recipe, substitute diced turnips for some or all of the potatoes; the flavor of turnips is a perfect match for potatoes. They take about 5 more minutes to cook than the potatoes, so if using both, add them first; simmer for 20 to 25 minutes total. When choosing turnips, select smaller ones since they are less bitter.

2 tablespoons regular olive oil

2¼ pounds lamb shoulder, finely diced

1 red onion, chopped

3 garlic cloves, chopped

Sea salt

Freshly ground black pepper

1 tablespoon tomato paste

1 quart (4 cups) chicken broth

½ pound baby red potatoes, quartered

1 (15-ounce) can white beans, drained and rinsed

2 tablespoons fresh thyme leaves

1. In a large pot, heat the oil over medium-high heat.

2. Add the lamb, and cook for 2 to 3 minutes per side, or until browned all over. Reduce the heat to medium, add the onion and garlic, and cook for 5 to 7 minutes, or until crisp-tender. Season with salt and pepper. Make room in the center, add the tomato paste, and cook for 1 minute.

3. Add the broth, bring to a boil, reduce to a simmer, and add the potatoes, beans, and thyme. Simmer for 15 to 20 minutes, or until the potatoes are tender and the stew is thickened.

4. Divide among 8 bowls, and serve hot.

PER SERVING CALORIES: 373 FAT: 14 G TOTAL CARBOHYDRATES: 17 G
DIETARY FIBER: 4 G SUGARS: 3 G PROTEIN: 42 G

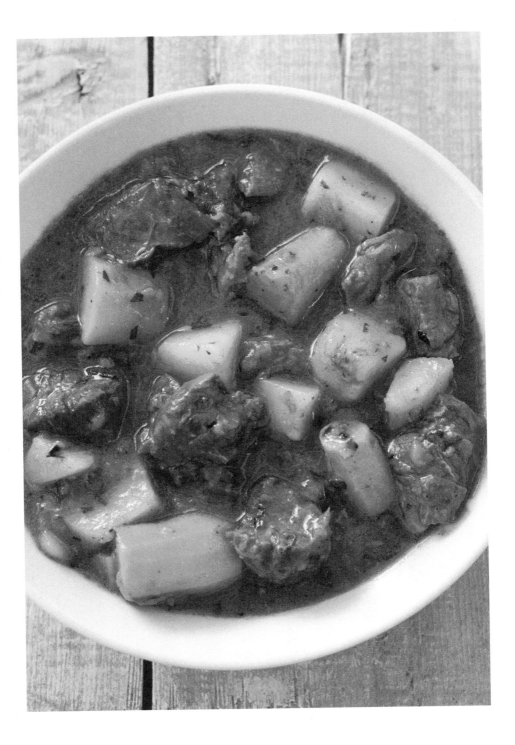

HEARTY BEEF STEW

Dairy-Free | Nut-Free | Paleo-Friendly

PREP TIME: 10 MINUTES ▲ COOK TIME: 35 MINUTES

SERVES 4   *Serve this nourishing stew on a bed of quinoa or with the Kale Caesar Salad (page 87) for a complete meal. If you want the beef extra tender, then cut the beef into half-inch cubes.*

....

Timesaving Tip: Whenever you have a lot of prep to perform, staying organized is key to being efficient. This is called mise en place *in restaurant kitchens, or "meez" for short. Place all your whole produce in one bowl and your prepped produce in additional bowls, grouping them according to when they will hit the pan.*

- **2 tablespoons regular olive oil**
- **1 pound beef chuck or top round, cut into 1-inch cubes**
- **1 red onion, chopped**
- **2 carrots, chopped**
- **2 celery stalks, chopped**
- **3 garlic cloves, chopped**
- **Sea salt**
- **Freshly ground black pepper**
- **1 tablespoon tomato paste**
- **1 quart (4 cups) beef broth**
- **1 pound Yukon Gold potatoes, peeled and quartered**
- **2 tablespoons fresh thyme leaves**

1. In a large pot, heat the oil over medium-high heat.

2. Add the beef, and cook for 2 to 3 minutes per side, or until browned all over. Reduce the heat to medium, add the onion, carrots, celery, and garlic, and cook for 5 to 7 minutes, or until crisp-tender. Season with salt and pepper. »

3. Make room in the center, add the tomato paste, and cook for 1 minute. Add the broth, bring to a boil, reduce to a simmer, and add the potatoes and thyme.

4. Simmer for 15 to 20 minutes, or until the potatoes are tender and the stew is thickened.

5. Divide among 4 bowls, and serve hot.

PER SERVING   CALORIES: 429   FAT: 16 G   TOTAL CARBOHYDRATES: 29 G
DIETARY FIBER: 4 G   SUGARS: 5 G   PROTEIN: 42 G

HEARTY SAUSAGE
AND BEAN STEW

Dairy-Free | Nut-Free

PREP TIME: 10 MINUTES ▲ TOTAL TIME: 35 MINUTES

SERVES 8   *This recipe calls for sweet Italian sausage, but feel free to substitute any kind of fresh sausage you like, such as chicken-apple sausage, kielbasa, or chorizo. Similarly, you can do the same with the beans.*

2 tablespoons regular olive oil

1 pound sweet Italian sausage, chopped

1 red onion, chopped

2 carrots, chopped

2 celery stalks, chopped

3 garlic cloves, chopped

Sea salt

Freshly ground black pepper

1 tablespoon tomato paste

1 quart (4 cups) beef broth

½ pound baby red potatoes, quartered

1 (15-ounce) can kidney beans, drained and rinsed

2 tablespoons chopped fresh rosemary leaves

1. In a large pot, heat the oil over medium-high heat.

2. Add the sausage, and cook for 5 minutes, or until browned all over. Reduce the heat to medium, add the onion, carrots, celery, and garlic, and cook for 5 to 7 minutes, or until crisp-tender. Season with salt and pepper. Make room in the center, add the tomato paste, and cook for 1 minute.

3. Add the broth, bring to a boil, reduce to a simmer, and add the potatoes, beans, and rosemary. Simmer for 15 to 20 minutes, or until the potatoes are tender and the stew is thickened.

PER SERVING   CALORIES: 351   FAT: 10 G   TOTAL CARBOHYDRATES: 43 G
DIETARY FIBER: 10 G   SUGARS: 3 G   PROTEIN: 25 G

PAN-ROASTED MOROCCAN-STYLE CHICKEN

Dairy-Free | Paleo-Friendly

PREP TIME: 5 MINUTES ▲ COOK TIME: 35 MINUTES

SERVES 4   *A tagine is a Moroccan dish of stewed meats cooked with spices, nuts, and dried fruits, and there are many regional variations of it. Tagine is also the name of the earthenware pot it is cooked in, with a cone-shaped lid and a hole at the top to allow the steam to escape at a controlled rate. This version shortens the long cooking time and eliminates the need to buy special equipment. Serve with Sautéed Swiss Chard with Raisins and Almonds (page 125).*

Diet Variation: To make this recipe nut-free, substitute ¼ cup pumpkin seeds for the almonds.

- **2 tablespoons regular olive oil**
- **1 pound bone-in, skin-on chicken thighs**
- **½ teaspoon ground coriander**
- **½ teaspoon ground turmeric**
- **½ teaspoon ground cumin**
- **½ teaspoon ground cinnamon**
- **Sea salt**
- **Freshly ground black pepper**
- **3 garlic cloves, chopped**
- **1 red onion, sliced**
- **¼ cup raisins**
- **¼ cup whole almonds, toasted**

1. Preheat the oven to 425°F.

2. In a large, ovenproof skillet, heat the oil over medium-high heat.

3. Season the chicken thighs with the coriander, turmeric, cumin, cinnamon, salt, and pepper. Add the chicken skin side down, and cook for 3 to 4 minutes, or until the skin is browned. Remove the chicken with tongs to a plate. Reduce the heat to medium, add the garlic and red onion, and cook for 5 to 7 minutes, or until the onion is crisp-tender.

4. Add the chicken back in, and transfer the pan to the oven. Roast for about 20 to 25 minutes, or until an instant-read thermometer inserted into the center without touching the bone reads 165°F.

5. Serve with the raisins and almonds sprinkled on top.

PER SERVING CALORIES: 355 FAT: 19 G TOTAL CARBOHYDRATES: 13 G
DIETARY FIBER: 2 G SUGARS: 7 G PROTEIN: 35 G

MEATBALLS WITH MARINARA SAUCE

Dairy-Free

PREP TIME: 15 MINUTES ▲ COOK TIME: 15 MINUTES

SERVES 4   *Pine nuts add a little extra texture to these hearty and satisfying meatballs. This version uses just beef, but feel free to substitute lamb, pork, or a combination of the three meats. If you want to give the dish a Sicilian twist, try adding half a cup of raisins or currants.*

1 pound ground beef

1 egg, beaten

½ cup finely chopped red onion

½ cup pine nuts, toasted

½ cup finely chopped fresh flat-leaf parsley

½ cup finely chopped fresh oregano

Sea salt

Freshly ground black pepper

2 tablespoons regular olive oil

½ cup Quick Marinara Sauce (page 272)

1. In a medium bowl, combine the beef, egg, onion, pine nuts, parsley, and oregano. Season with salt and pepper.

2. Form loosely into 1½-inch balls.

3. In a large skillet, heat the oil over medium-high heat. Add the meatballs in a single layer (you may need to do this in batches), and cook for about 10 minutes, turning them occasionally, or until browned on all sides and an instant-read thermometer inserted into the center of a meatball reads 160°F.

4. Serve with the Quick Marinara Sauce on the side.

PER SERVING   CALORIES: 464   FAT: 30 G   TOTAL CARBOHYDRATES: 14 G
DIETARY FIBER: 6 G   SUGARS: 4 G   PROTEIN: 40 G

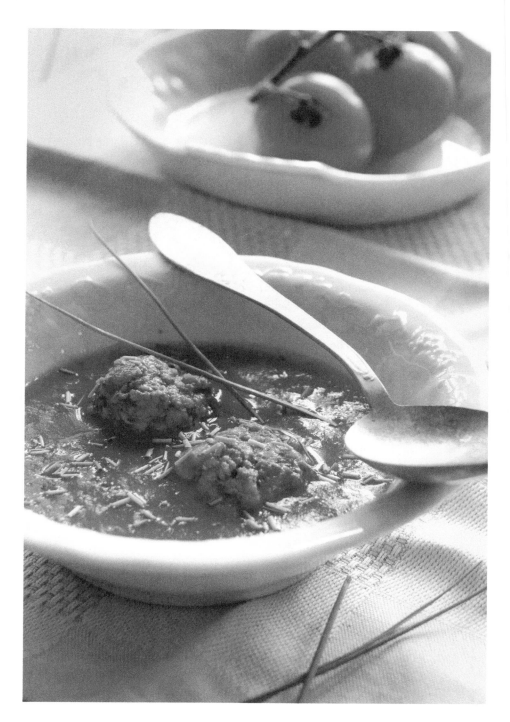

THAI STREET CHICKEN

Dairy-Free | Nut-Free | Paleo-Friendly

SERVES 6   *In Thailand, whole chickens are marinated, and then grilled and served with a tamarind-based sauce. To make a simpler version of chicken gai yang, skin-on chicken breasts and thighs are used. Since tamarind can be difficult to find, a citrus-honey glaze is brushed on the chicken.*

Timesaving Tip: To make quick work of peeling garlic, peel the outer layer of skin off each head to reveal the cloves, place both your palms over the head, and press down with all your body weight. This should break the head into separate cloves. Then, place in a mixing bowl, and place another mixing bowl on top, upside down. Shake vigorously to loosen the skins.

- 3 lemongrass stalks
- 1 tablespoon fish sauce
- Juice of 2 limes, divided
- 2 tablespoons honey, divided
- 10 sprigs cilantro
- 2 tablespoons black peppercorns
- 3 serrano chiles, stemmed and chopped
- 2 garlic heads, peeled
- 2 (4-ounce) skin-on, boneless chicken breasts
- 4 skin-on, boneless chicken thighs
- 2 teaspoons ground turmeric
- 2 teaspoons ground coriander

1. Remove and discard the tough outer layers of the lemongrass stalks, and thinly slice the tender core.

2. In the bowl of a food processor, place the lemongrass, fish sauce, juice of 1 lime, 1 tablespoon honey, cilantro, peppercorns, chiles, and garlic, and process until combined. Rub the marinade over the chicken breasts, and marinate for at least 1 hour (overnight is better).

3. When you are ready to cook, prepare a gas or charcoal grill for high-heat cooking.

4. Shake excess marinade off the chicken breasts and discard the marinade. Season the chicken thighs with the turmeric and coriander, and place the chicken breasts and thighs on the grill.

5. In a small bowl, stir together the remaining juice of 1 lime and 1 tablespoon honey.

6. Grill the breasts for 3 to 4 minutes per side and the chicken thighs for 5 to 7 minutes per side, brushing occasionally with the glaze, or until an instant-read thermometer inserted into the center reads 165°F.

PER SERVING CALORIES: 335 FAT: 11 G TOTAL CARBOHYDRATES: 15 G
DIETARY FIBER: 2 G SUGARS: 6 G PROTEIN: 44 G

EASY ROAST CHICKEN WITH ROSEMARY AND GARLIC

Dairy-Free | Nut-Free | Paleo-Friendly

PREP TIME: 5 MINUTES ▲ COOK TIME: 20 MINUTES

SERVES 6   *To have roast chicken for leftovers during the week, ask the butcher to cut the chicken into eighths. This way, you can make Chicken Salad with Garlic Aïoli (page 84) later in the week.*

Ingredient Tip: Because of the way most chickens are processed, they can contain up to 5 percent water by weight. This means you're paying for the water and also for less flavorful, soggy meat. For a more "chicken-y" chicken, look for air-chilled chicken, which has more flavor, better texture, and no retained water.

1 whole chicken, cut into 8 pieces

2 tablespoons regular olive oil

Sea salt

Freshly ground black pepper

2 tablespoons chopped rosemary

1 head garlic, cut in half

1. Preheat the oven to 450°F.

2. Coat the chicken with the oil, and season with salt and pepper. Place the chicken skin side up in a baking dish, top with the rosemary and rub all over with the cut side of the garlic. Transfer the dish to the oven.

3. Roast the chicken for 20 minutes, or until an instant-read thermometer inserted into the center without touching the bone reads 165°F.

PER SERVING   CALORIES: 590   FAT: 32 G   TOTAL CARBOHYDRATES: 2 G
DIETARY FIBER: 1 G   SUGARS: 0 G   PROTEIN: 60 G

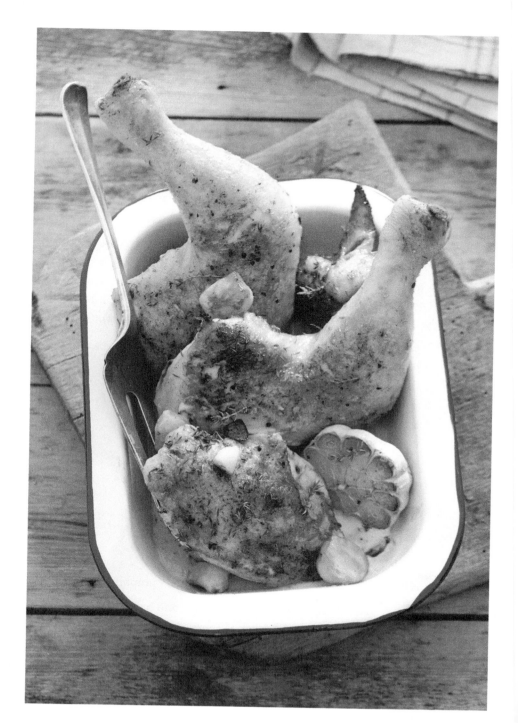

PUMPKIN SEED–CRUSTED CHICKEN WITH EASY PICO DE GALLO

Dairy-Free | Nut-Free | Paleo-Friendly

PREP TIME: 5 MINUTES ▲ COOK TIME: 30 MINUTES

SERVES 4   *For an easy weeknight chicken dish with a Mexican flair, look no further than this simple recipe. By using nutty pumpkin seeds as a coating, there's no need to use panko or breadcrumbs to give chicken breasts a juicy, moist interior and a nice exterior crust. In addition to their wonderful flavor, pumpkin seeds add a good dose of protein, fiber, and vitamin K to the dish. To complete the meal, try serving with some Mexican Grilled Corn (page 117).*

4 (4-ounce) boneless, skinless chicken breasts

1 teaspoon ground cumin

Sea salt

Freshly ground black pepper

1 cup pepitas or shelled pumpkin seeds, chopped

1 egg, beaten

1 cup Easy Pico de Gallo (page 270)

1. Preheat the oven to 350°F.

2. Season the chicken with the cumin, salt, and pepper.

3. Place the pumpkin seeds on a plate.

4. Dredge the chicken in the egg, followed by the pumpkin seeds.

5. Transfer to a baking dish, place in the oven, and bake for 30 minutes, or until an instant-read thermometer reads 165°F.

6. Serve the chicken with the Easy Pico de Gallo on top.

PER SERVING   CALORIES: 418   FAT: 25 G   TOTAL CARBOHYDRATES: 10 G
DIETARY FIBER: 2 G   SUGARS: 1 G   PROTEIN: 43 G

ALMOND-CRUSTED CHICKEN WITH BUTTERMILK DRESSING

PREP TIME: 5 MINUTES ▲ COOK TIME: 30 MINUTES

SERVES 4   *Almond meal is the best grain-free replacement for bread-crumbs. It's available online and at most grocery stores (Bob's Red Mill is a good brand to try). The crisp chicken is topped with Buttermilk Dressing. Red Wine–Braised Red Cabbage (page 131) makes the perfect side.*

1 egg
½ cup almond meal
Sea salt
Freshly ground black pepper
4 (4-ounce) boneless, skinless chicken breasts
2 tablespoons regular olive oil
¼ cup Buttermilk Dressing (page 289)

1. Preheat the oven to 350°F.

2. Beat the egg in a shallow dish. Spread the almond meal on a second shallow dish. Season generously with salt and pepper.

3. Dredge the chicken in the egg, followed by the almond meal.

4. Coat a baking dish with the oil. Arrange the chicken in a single layer in the baking dish. Bake for 30 minutes, or until an instant-read thermometer reads 165°F.

5. Divide the chicken among 4 plates. Serve with the Buttermilk Dressing drizzled on top.

PER SERVING   CALORIES: 443   FAT: 32 G   TOTAL CARBOHYDRATES: 3 G
DIETARY FIBER: 2 G   SUGARS: 1 G   PROTEIN: 37 G

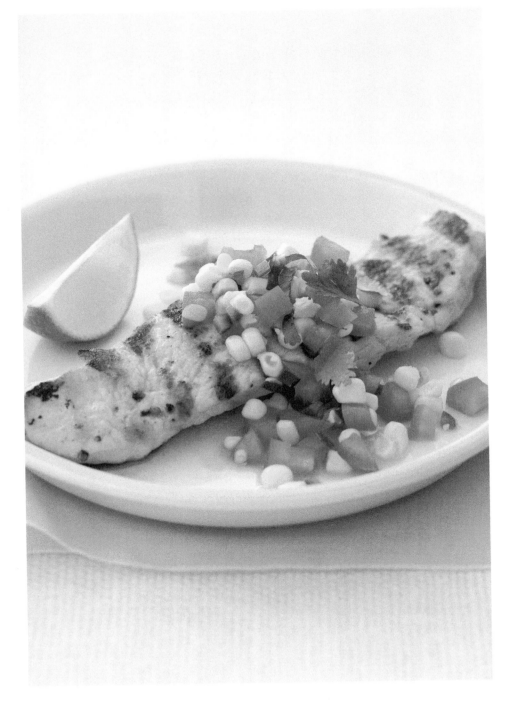

GRILLED PORK TENDERLOIN WITH CORN AND TOMATO

Dairy-Free | Nut-Free | Paleo-Friendly

PREP TIME: 5 MINUTES ▲ COOK TIME: 30 MINUTES

SERVES 4   *Short on time and need to get dinner on the table in a flash? This Southwestern-inspired pork dish can be ready in just 30 minutes or so. Whip up a quick side like Sautéed Swiss Chard with Raisins and Almonds (page 125) as the pork cooks on the grill.*

> 2 tablespoons regular olive oil
>
> 1 pound pork tenderloin, cut lengthwise into strips
>
> Sea salt
>
> Freshly ground black pepper
>
> ½ cup corn kernels, thawed if frozen
>
> ½ cup chopped tomatoes
>
> 1 tablespoon cilantro leaves, for garnish (optional)

1. Prepare a gas or charcoal grill for medium-heat cooking.

2. Brush the grill with olive oil. Season the pork with the salt and pepper. Add the pork, and grill, covered, for 12 to 15 minutes, or until an instant-read thermometer inserted into the thickest part reads 140°F. Turn the tenderloin every 2 minutes. Let the pork cool at least 5 minutes before slicing lengthwise.

3. Top the pork with the corn and tomatoes, and garnish with cilantro (if using).

PER SERVING CALORIES: 241 FAT: 11 G TOTAL CARBOHYDRATES: 5 G
DIETARY FIBER: 1 G SUGARS: 1 G PROTEIN: 30 G

CHICKEN CACCIATORE

Nut-Free | Dairy-Free | Paleo-Friendly

PREP TIME: 10 MINUTES ▲ COOK TIME: 35 MINUTES

SERVES 4   *Chicken cacciatore, or hunter's-style chicken, is an Italian stew simmered in tomato sauce with white wine and capers. If you're looking for a one-pot meal, consider this dish. For an interesting variation, try making this with veal loin or rib chops instead. Serve with Pugliese-Style Broccoli Rabe (page 113) for a complete Italian meal.*

- 2 tablespoons regular olive oil
- 1 pound bone-in, skin-on chicken thighs
- Sea salt
- Freshly ground black pepper
- 1 teaspoon capers, drained and rinsed
- ½ red onion, chopped
- 2 carrots, chopped
- 2 celery stalks, chopped
- 1 cup white wine
- 1 cup Quick Marinara Sauce (page 272)
- ¼ cup finely chopped fresh flat-leaf parsley

1. Preheat the oven to 425°F.

2. In a large, ovenproof skillet with a lid, heat the oil over high heat. Season the chicken with salt and pepper, and place in the skillet skin side down. Cook for 3 to 4 minutes, or until the skin is browned. Using tongs, remove the chicken to a plate.

3. Add the capers, onion, carrots, and celery to the skillet. Cook for 5 to 7 minutes, or until crisp-tender, then add the white wine and boil until the sauce is reduced by half.

4. Add the chicken back in, top with the Quick Marinara Sauce, transfer the pan to the oven, and cook, covered, for about 20 to 25 minutes.

5. Divide the chicken, vegetables, and sauce among 4 bowls. Top with the parsley before serving.

PER SERVING   CALORIES: 400   FAT: 19 G   TOTAL CARBOHYDRATES: 12 G
DIETARY FIBER: 3 G   SUGARS: 6 G   PROTEIN: 35 G

CRISP DUCK BREAST WITH HOMEMADE PEANUT SAUCE

Dairy-Free | Paleo-Friendly

PREP TIME: 5 MINUTES ▲ COOK TIME: 30 MINUTES

SERVES 2   *Perfectly seared duck breasts with crispy skin and just the tiniest layer of fat underneath may seem like the realm of fancy French restaurants, but it's actually a simple feat to pull off, as long as you know a couple of tricks. The duck breasts are cooked to medium rare and served with a delicious Homemade Peanut Sauce (page 292), which you can make as the breasts slowly render out their fat. Serve with a side of greens like Sautéed Spinach with Nutmeg (page 119).*

Cooking Tip: Searing duck breasts will result in a fair amount of rendered fat, but don't throw it out. Instead, once cool, strain the duck fat through a colander, transfer to containers, and freeze for later use. It's great for frying eggs sunny side up for breakfast, or adding rich flavor to a side of Roasted Rosemary Potatoes (page 135).

2 skin-on, boneless duck breasts

2 tablespoons chopped scallions, white and green parts, for garnish

¼ cup Homemade Peanut Sauce (page 292)

1. Heat a large skillet over high heat until smoking hot.

2. Score the skin on the duck breasts at a 45-degree angle, making slits through the skin every half inch or so and taking care not to pierce through to the meat underneath (this will cause the meat to dry out as it cooks).

3. Place the breasts skin side down, and cook undisturbed for about 5 minutes, or until the skin is browned and crisp. Reduce the heat to low, and cook until the fat between the skin and meat shrinks to a thin layer. Keeping one hand on the meat, carefully pour off the fat into a nonreactive container periodically.

4. Using tongs, flip the breasts and cook for 4 to 6 more minutes for medium rare.

5. Garnish with the scallions and serve with the Homemade Peanut Sauce.

PER SERVING   CALORIES: 281   FAT: 11 G   TOTAL CARBOHYDRATES: 4 G
DIETARY FIBER: 1 G   SUGARS: 3 G   PROTEIN: 40 G

CHAPTER 11

Sweets and Treats

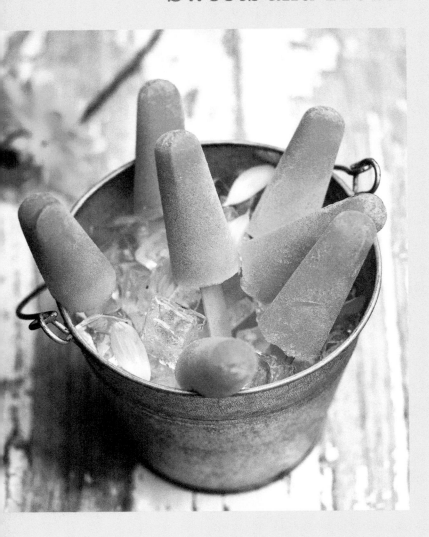

CHOCOLATE-VANILLA SHAKE

Nut-Free | Vegetarian

PREP TIME: 5 MINUTES

SERVES 2 *Chocolate lovers, rejoice! Your milkshake has arrived. Rich with the flavor of homemade chocolate sauce made with semisweet chocolate chips, this shake is one you'll have a hard time sharing. For even more intense flavor, feel free to add more chocolate sauce.*

3 scoops Honey–Vanilla Bean Ice Cream (page 243)

½ cup Chocolate Sauce (page 293)

½ cup milk

In a blender, process the Honey–Vanilla Bean Ice Cream, Chocolate Sauce, and milk until smooth. Divide into tall glasses and serve.

PER SERVING   CALORIES: 493   FAT: 33 G   TOTAL CARBOHYDRATES: 48 G
DIETARY FIBER: 2 G   SUGARS: 40 G   PROTEIN: 5 G

STRAWBERRY SHAKE

Nut-Free | Vegetarian

PREP TIME: 5 MINUTES

SERVES 2   *Summer never felt so fine. This strawberry milkshake features real fruit and honey. If you prefer a smoother shake, you can strain the Strawberry Coulis first through a fine-mesh strainer before adding it to the mix.*

3 scoops Honey–Vanilla Bean Ice Cream (page 243)
½ cup Strawberry Coulis (page 294)
½ cup milk

In a blender, process the Honey–Vanilla Bean Ice Cream, Strawberry Coulis, and milk until smooth. Divide into tall glasses and serve.

PER SERVING   CALORIES: 599   FAT: 38 G   TOTAL CARBOHYDRATES: 60 G
DIETARY FIBER: 2 G   SUGARS: 53 G   PROTEIN: 11 G

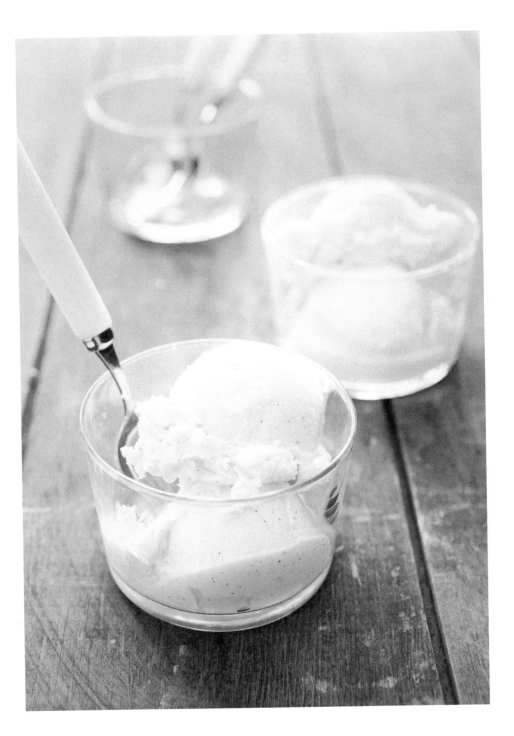

HONEY–VANILLA BEAN
ICE CREAM

Nut-Free

PREP TIME: 5 MINUTES (PLUS FREEZING TIME) ▲ COOK TIME: 20 MINUTES

SERVES 16   *Using tempered eggs and a strained custard, this is the old-fashioned French way of making ice cream. No vanilla ice cream recipe can compare to the rich flavor of one with an egg-based custard. Feel free to experiment with mix-ins like chocolate chips or nuts; add them in just before freezing.*

Cooking Tip: Making the custard for this ice cream can't be rushed. You may be tempted to turn up the heat to speed up the process (and perhaps relieve yourself from some stirring) but that will cause the eggs to scramble, and you'll have to start over.

- 2 pints milk
- 2 pints heavy cream
- 7 ounces honey, divided
- 1 vanilla bean, split
- 5 egg yolks

1. In a medium pot, bring the milk, heavy cream, and 3½ ounces of honey to a simmer.

2. Scrape the seeds from the vanilla bean into the pot, and add the bean to the pot. Turn off the heat and let sit for 20 minutes.

3. Meanwhile, in a medium bowl, beat the egg yolks with the remaining 3½ ounces of honey.

4. Temper the egg yolks by adding half of the milk mixture to the eggs and stirring, then return the eggs and milk to the pot. »

5. Cook the egg-milk mixture over low heat, stirring continuously with a wooden spoon, making sure to stir along the edges of the pot as well as the center, until thickened. The mixture is thick enough when a finger drawn across the back of the spoon leaves a clean streak.

6. Strain through a colander into a bowl, and place that bowl into another bowl filled with ice. Transfer to the refrigerator once cooled.

7. Process in an ice cream machine according to the manufacturer's directions, transfer to containers, and freeze for at least 1 hour, or until set.

PER SERVING CALORIES: 293 FAT: 25 G TOTAL CARBOHYDRATES: 15 G
DIETARY FIBER: 0 G SUGARS: 13 G PROTEIN: 4 G

HONEY–VANILLA BEAN SHAKE

Nut-Free | Vegetarian

PREP TIME: 5 MINUTES

SERVES 2   *If you've already learned how to make your own ice cream using the Honey–Vanilla Bean Ice Cream recipe (page 243), then you're only one step away from making your own shakes, too. Start with this basic yet delicious recipe. All you need to do is add milk, blend, and enjoy! Add your favorite mix-ins like chopped nuts and whipped cream to go over the top.*

If you're thinking of using store-bought ice cream, proceed with caution. Although it will save you some time, most ice creams contain hidden sources of gluten. They usually fall under the guise of "natural flavorings" on the ingredients list. If you do decide to use store-bought ice cream, choose the brand with the shortest ingredients list and ingredients with recognizable names. Vanilla ice cream, for example, should only contain cream, milk, sugar, egg yolks, and vanilla beans or vanilla extract.

3 scoops Honey–Vanilla Bean Ice Cream (page 243)
½ cup milk

In a blender, process the Honey–Vanilla Bean Ice Cream and milk until smooth. Divide into tall glasses and serve

PER SERVING   CALORIES: 478   FAT: 38 G   TOTAL CARBOHYDRATES: 28 G
DIETARY FIBER: 0 G   SUGARS: 24 G   PROTEIN: 10 G

FLAN

Nut-Free

PREP TIME: 5 MINUTES ▲ COOK TIME: 40 MINUTES
COOLING TIME: 6 HOURS

SERVES 6   *Flan, the classic Spanish dessert, is a sweet custard that's dense and rich, with just a hint of vanilla and cinnamon. For an interesting variation, try substituting almond extract for the vanilla bean.*

Cooking Tip: A pair of sturdy metal tongs is the easiest way to handle hot ramekins from the oven.

- 1 pint milk
- 1 teaspoon ground cinnamon
- ½ vanilla bean, split and scraped
- 3 egg yolks
- 3 tablespoons honey

1. Preheat the oven to 325°F, and position a rack in the center.

2. In a medium pot, bring the milk, cinnamon, and vanilla to a boil.

3. Meanwhile, in a medium bowl, beat the egg yolks with the honey.

4. Add half of the milk mixture to the eggs and stir, then strain the remaining half of the milk mixture into the bowl.

5. Transfer to the ramekins, and place the ramekins in a baking dish. Place the baking dish on the center rack of the oven, and carefully fill with enough hot water to come halfway up the sides of the ramekins. Bake for 35 to 40 minutes, or until the center of each custard no longer jiggles when shaken.

6. Using tongs, remove each ramekin from the baking dish. Cool at room temperature for 30 minutes, then cover and refrigerate until set, about 4 to 6 hours.

PER SERVING CALORIES: 107   FAT: 4 G   TOTAL CARBOHYDRATES: 14 G
DIETARY FIBER: 0 G   SUGARS: 13 G   PROTEIN: 6 G

BANANA SPLIT

Vegetarian

PREP TIME: 5 MINUTES

SERVES 2 *What better way to celebrate making your own ice cream—
Honey–Vanilla Bean Ice Cream (page 243)—than with a banana split you
can share with a friend? This version is topped with homemade Chocolate
Sauce (page 293), toasted almonds, and of course, a cherry.*

*Diet Variation: To make this nut-free, omit the almonds and substitute
chocolate chips instead.*

3 scoops Honey–Vanilla Bean Ice Cream (page 243)

1 ripe banana, spilt lengthwise

¼ cup sliced almonds, toasted

1 tablespoon Chocolate Sauce (page 293)

1 cherry

1. Scoop the Honey–Vanilla Bean Ice Cream into a shallow dish.

2. Arrange the banana slices on either side.

3. Top with the almonds, Chocolate Sauce, and cherry.

PER SERVING CALORIES: 364 FAT: 25 G TOTAL CARBOHYDRATES: 32 G
DIETARY FIBER: 4 G SUGARS: 21 G PROTEIN: 6 G

HONEY-CHOCOLATE
MOUSSE

Nut-Free

PREP TIME: 20 MINUTES (PLUS REFRIGERATION TIME)

COOK TIME: 10 MINUTES

SERVES 4   *Light and airy, the magic of chocolate mousse lies in the power of egg whites that turn fluffy when beaten. Make sure to use the freshest eggs for this recipe since they remain uncooked, or use pasteurized eggs. For a flavor twist, try adding various flavorings, such as chopped rosemary or chili powder.*

Cooking Tip: Do not allow water to come into contact with any of the melted chocolate for this recipe, or it will harden and become impossible to work with, a condition known as "seizing."

- 5 ounces semisweet chocolate
- 1½ cups heavy cream
- 3 egg whites
- 1½ tablespoons honey
- 1 teaspoon vanilla extract

1. Bring 1 inch of water to a simmer in a medium pot, and place a bowl snugly over the top. Add the chocolate and melt, stirring occasionally with a spatula, then turn off the heat once it is melted completely.

2. Place the cream in a small bowl, and place the bowl inside of another larger bowl filled with ice.

3. Using a whisk, beat the cream until it thickens; the cream should just curl over softly when the whisk is held upright. Place in the refrigerator. »

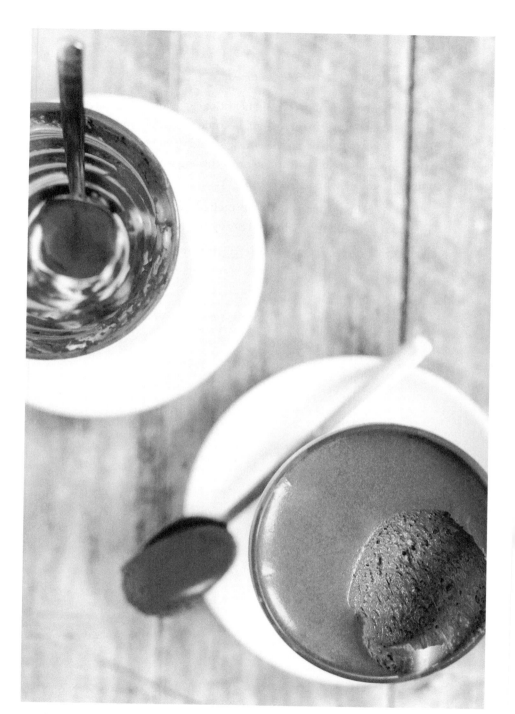

4. In another bowl, using a whisk, beat the egg whites until they increase in volume, foam up, and become stiff. They should also just curl over softly when the whisk is held upright. While still whisking, slowly add the honey until the egg whites curl over stiffly when the whisk is held upright.

5. Whisk ¼ of the egg whites into the melted chocolate, fold the rest in, and then fold in the whipped heavy cream and vanilla extract.

6. Pour into 4 serving bowls, and refrigerate for about 1 hour, or until set.

PER SERVING CALORIES: 364 FAT: 27 G TOTAL CARBOHYDRATES: 30 G
DIETARY FIBER: 2 G SUGARS: 26 G PROTEIN: 5 G

CHOCOLATE EGG CREAM

Nut-Free | Vegetarian

PREP TIME: 5 MINUTES

SERVES 1   *People who have never had an egg cream assume that there must be cream and eggs in this drink, but they're in for a surprise. Why? Because it has neither. A chocolate egg cream has just three ingredients: soda, milk, and syrup. This version uses a homemade Chocolate Sauce (page 293), but you can substitute your favorite brand (as long as it's grain-free, of course).*

Diet Variation: To make this dairy-free, substitute almond milk in the drink and in the Chocolate Sauce.

½ cup milk

½ cup club soda

2 tablespoons Chocolate Sauce (page 293)

Fill a chilled glass with the milk, followed by the club soda and Chocolate Sauce, and mix vigorously.

PER SERVING   CALORIES: 374   FAT: 19 G   TOTAL CARBOHYDRATES: 50 G
DIETARY FIBER: 0 G   SUGARS: 30 G   PROTEIN: 6 G

CHOCOLATE-CHILI BROWNIES

SERVES 8 *Chocolate and chili powder may seem like an unusual combination, but in Mexico, it's one that figures prominently in the cuisine. There, it's not unusual to see the two together in sauces, drinks, and desserts. This unique flavor combination was the inspiration behind these Chocolate-Chili Brownies. For an interesting twist, try using different types of chili powder such as ancho chili powder.*

   6 tablespoons unsalted butter, softened, plus more for the baking dish

   12 ounces semisweet chocolate chips

   ⅓ cup honey

   1 teaspoon chili powder

   2 eggs, at room temperature

   3 tablespoons almond flour

   3 tablespoons coconut flour

   1 teaspoon salt

   1 teaspoon baking powder

1. Preheat the oven to 325°F, and grease an 8-by-8-inch baking dish with butter.

2. Bring 1 inch of water to a simmer in a medium pot, and place a bowl snugly over the top. Add the chocolate to the bowl and melt it, stirring occasionally with a spatula.

3. Meanwhile, using an electric mixer, cream the butter and honey together on medium speed until smooth, about 3 minutes. Add the melted chocolate and chili powder to the butter, and beat on medium speed until incorporated. Add the eggs one at a time, making sure to mix well each time.

4. In another bowl, whisk together the almond and coconut flours, salt, and baking powder, and slowly add the flour mixture to the wet mixture, mixing on low speed until just incorporated.

5. Fill the baking dish with the mixture, and bake until a toothpick inserted into the center of the brownies comes out clean, about 20 minutes. Let cool on a wire rack until completely cool, then cut into 8 pieces.

PER SERVING   CALORIES: 418   FAT: 27 G   TOTAL CARBOHYDRATES: 43 G
DIETARY FIBER: 5 G   SUGARS: 33 G   PROTEIN: 4 G

BLACKBERRY LASSI

Nut-Free | Vegetarian

PREP TIME: 5 MINUTES

SERVES 1   *Lassi, a yogurt-based drink from India, is popular there on hot summer days. It is made with the leftover liquid from straining yogurt, but this version uses store-bought buttermilk, which has a similar flavor. The addition of cardamom lends a particularly exotic dessert element to this drink. Feel free to experiment with other fruit like mangoes or raspberries. Serve this for dessert to cool down after a spicy meal like South Indian–Style Fish Curry (page 191).*

Diet Variation: To make this vegan, use almond milk instead of the buttermilk and pure agave instead of the honey.

    6 ounces fresh blackberries
    ¼ teaspoon ground cardamom
    1 cup buttermilk
    1 tablespoon honey

1. Place the blackberries, cardamom, buttermilk, and honey in a blender or the bowl of a food processor, and process until the mixture reaches a smoothie-like consistency.

2. If you wish, strain out the seeds using a fine-mesh strainer. Pour into a glass.

PER SERVING   CALORIES: 237   FAT: 3 G   TOTAL CARBOHYDRATES: 46 G
DIETARY FIBER: 9 G   SUGARS: 37 G   PROTEIN: 11 G

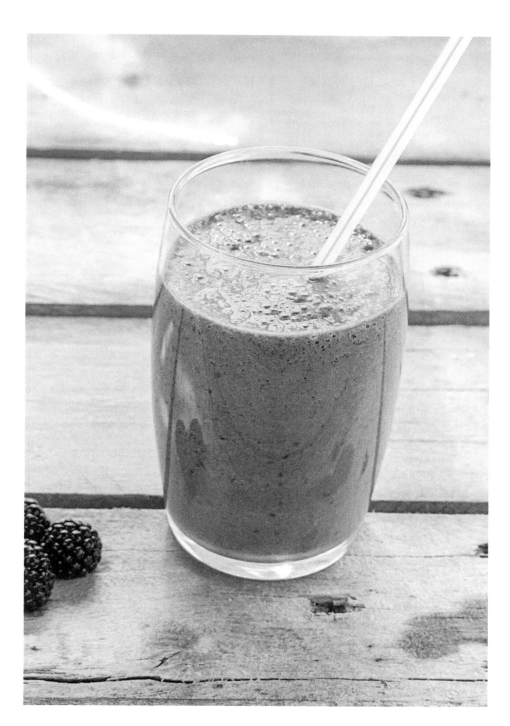

HONEY SNICKERDOODLES

SERVES 12   *The cinnamon-laced aroma of snickerdoodles wafting through the kitchen as they bake in the oven is unmistakable. This version uses honey instead of refined brown sugar, making it diet-friendly. If you like, add a few grinds of nutmeg to the batter.*

½ cup unsalted butter, at room temperature

1½ cups honey

1 egg

1 teaspoon vanilla extract

¾ cup almond flour

¼ cup coconut flour

1 teaspoon baking soda

2 teaspoons ground cinnamon

1. Preheat the oven to 375°F. Line a baking sheet with parchment paper.

2. In a large bowl, cream the butter and the honey together using an electric mixer on low speed until smooth, about 5 minutes. Add the egg and vanilla extract and mix until well incorporated.

3. Sift the almond and coconut flours into a separate bowl, add the baking soda and cinnamon, and stir to combine.

4. With the mixer on low speed, slowly add the flour mixture to the wet mixture. Blend until well incorporated, about 5 minutes.

5. Drop 1-tablespoon dollops of the dough 2 inches apart on the prepared baking sheet. Place in the oven and bake for about 15 minutes. Remove from the oven and let cool on a wire rack. Store the snickerdoodles in a cookie jar to keep moist.

PER SERVING   CALORIES: 224   FAT: 9 G   TOTAL CARBOHYDRATES: 37 G
DIETARY FIBER: 1 G   SUGARS: 35 G   PROTEIN: 1 G

BLONDIES

SERVES 8   *Blondies have semisweet chocolate chips distributed through-out the vanilla batter. Serve with a glass of milk for dipping.*

- **6 tablespoons unsalted butter, softened, plus more for the baking dish**
- **⅓ cup honey**
- **1 teaspoon pure vanilla extract**
- **2 eggs, at room temperature**
- **3 tablespoons almond flour**
- **3 tablespoons coconut flour**
- **1 teaspoon salt**
- **1 teaspoon baking powder**
- **6 ounces semisweet chocolate chips**

1. Preheat the oven to 325°F, and grease an 8-by-8-inch baking dish with butter.

2. Using an electric mixer, cream the butter and honey together on medium speed until smooth, about 3 minutes.

3. Add the vanilla extract, and beat on medium speed until incorporated.

4. Add the eggs one at a time, making sure to mix well each time.

5. In another bowl, whisk together the almond and coconut flours, salt, and baking powder, and slowly add the flour mixture to the wet mixture, mixing on low speed until just incorporated.

6. Stir in the chocolate chips.

7. Fill the baking dish with the mixture, and bake until a toothpick inserted into the center of the blondies comes out clean, about 20 minutes. Let cool on a wire rack until completely cool, then cut into 8 pieces.

PER SERVING   CALORIES: 314   FAT: 21 G   TOTAL CARBOHYDRATES: 29 G
DIETARY FIBER: 3 G   SUGARS: 23 G   PROTEIN: 4 G

HONEY PANNA COTTA

Nut-Free

SERVES 6   Panna cotta, *which means "cooked cream" in Italian, is a cold custard often flavored with vanilla, chocolate, or fruit. Here, it is flavored with real vanilla bean and sweetened with honey. Panna cotta is a bit similar to crème brûlée, the popular French dessert with caramelized sugar on top, but it has a firmer texture that's closer to flan and isn't quite as rich. It's the perfect ending to a lovely Italian meal.*

- **3 cups milk, divided**
- **1 (¼-ounce) packet gelatin**
- **½ cup honey**
- **1 vanilla bean, split and scraped**
- **2 ripe apricots, cut into small wedges, for garnish (optional)**
- **2 strawberries, cut into small wedges, for garnish (optional)**

1. In a small bowl, combine ½ cup milk with the gelatin, and set aside for 2 to 3 minutes to bloom.

2. Meanwhile, in a medium pot, heat the remaining 2½ cups of milk with the honey and vanilla until it comes to a boil. Watch it carefully.

3. Add the gelatin-and-milk mixture, and cook for 1 minute, stirring constantly.

4. Transfer the mixture to a medium mixing bowl, and place the bowl inside a large mixing bowl filled with ice.

5. When cool, transfer to ramekins, and place in the refrigerator for at least 4 hours, or until set. Garnish with the apricots and strawberries (if using).

PER SERVING   CALORIES: 153   FAT: 3 G   TOTAL CARBOHYDRATES: 30 G
DIETARY FIBER: 0 G   SUGARS: 29 G   PROTEIN: 5 G

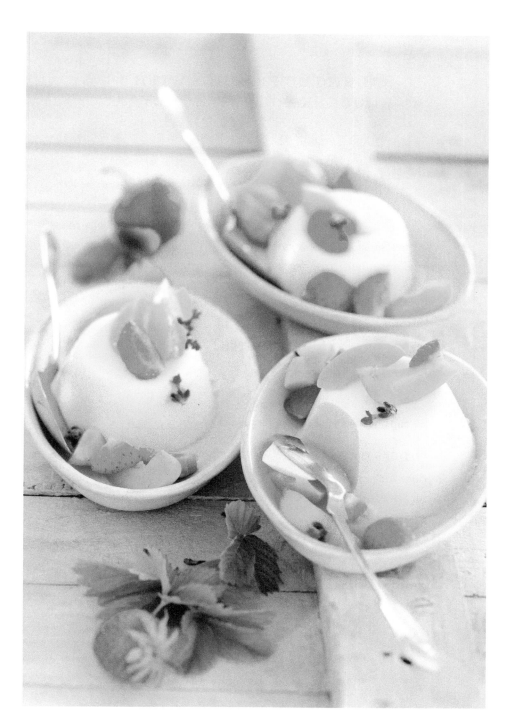

GRILLED PEACHES WITH GREEK YOGURT, HONEY, AND MINT

Nut-Free | Vegetarian

PREP TIME: 5 MINUTES ▲ COOK TIME: 10 MINUTES

SERVES 4   *Sometimes, the simplest things in life are best, like these grilled peaches with Greek yogurt and honey. While few things can compare to the allure of juicy, ripe peaches eaten in the summer, grilling them further enhances their sweetness. The natural sugars of the fruit caramelize when exposed to the heat of the grill. Serve with a fruity dessert wine such as moscato.*

> 1 pound ripe peaches, halved and pitted
>
> 1 tablespoon regular olive oil
>
> 1 tablespoon honey
>
> ½ cup nonfat plain Greek yogurt
>
> ¼ cup chopped mint leaves, for garnish

1. Prepare a gas or charcoal grill for medium-high-heat grilling.

2. Coat the peaches with the oil, and place on the grill cut side down for 5 minutes, or until grill marks appear. Turn and grill the other side for 2 to 3 minutes.

3. Meanwhile, in a small bowl, stir the honey into the yogurt.

4. Serve the peaches topped with a dollop of the yogurt and garnished with the mint leaves.

PER SERVING CALORIES: 108 FAT: 4 G TOTAL CARBOHYDRATES: 18 G
DIETARY FIBER: 3 G SUGARS: 16 G PROTEIN: 3 G

WATERMELON-JALAPEÑO
ICE POPS

Dairy-Free | Nut-Free | Paleo-Friendly | Vegetarian

PREP TIME: 5 MINUTES (PLUS REFRIGERATION AND FREEZING TIME)
COOK TIME: 5 MINUTES

SERVES 8   *These watermelon ice pops are made with some jalapeño pepper to create an icy-hot contrast. When choosing the watermelon, pick one that is firm and heavy for its size with a pale section on the rind, a sign of sweetness. For a variation, make these pops with honeydew.*

Warning: When working with hot peppers, avoid touching other parts of your body, especially your eyes. It's also a good idea to wear gloves when working with very hot peppers like habañeros. Hot peppers contain capsaicin, a compound that is responsible for the sensation of heat when you eat one.

⅓ cup honey

1 cup water

2 cups strained fresh watermelon juice

1 tablespoon finely chopped jalapeño pepper

1. In a small pot, combine the honey and water, bring to a boil, and cook until the honey dissolves. Transfer to a bowl, and place in the refrigerator for 30 minutes.

2. Stir in the watermelon juice and jalapeño, transfer to ice pop molds, and freeze according to the manufacturer's directions.

PER SERVING   CALORIES: 63   FAT: 0 G   TOTAL CARBOHYDRATES: 17 G
DIETARY FIBER: 0 G   SUGARS: 16 G   PROTEIN: 0 G

RASPBERRY-LIME ICE POPS WITH MINT

Dairy-Free | Nut-Free | Paleo-Friendly | Vegetarian

PREP TIME: 5 MINUTES (PLUS REFRIGERATION AND FREEZING TIME)
COOK TIME: 5 MINUTES

SERVES 8   *Here's a guilt-free, low-calorie treat that you can make together with the kids. The flavors of raspberry and lime complement each other nicely, and the mint adds to the cool factor. Make these ice pops when raspberries are at their peak in the summer. If using frozen raspberries, double the amount of honey.*

2 cups fresh raspberries

⅓ cup honey

1 cup water

1 tablespoon finely chopped mint

Juice of 1 lime

1. Purée the raspberries in a blender and set aside.

2. In a small pot, combine the honey and water, bring to a boil, and cook until the honey dissolves.

3. Transfer to a bowl, and place in the refrigerator for 30 minutes.

4. Stir in the blended raspberries, mint, and lime, and transfer to ice pop molds, and freeze according to the manufacturer's directions.

PER SERVING   CALORIES: 62   FAT: 0 G   TOTAL CARBOHYDRATES: 16 G
DIETARY FIBER: 2 G   SUGARS: 13 G   PROTEIN: 1 G

BERRIES WITH FRESH WHIPPED CREAM AND MINT

Nut-Free | Vegetarian

PREP TIME: 10 MINUTES

SERVES 4   *A no-fuss classic dessert gets a bit of a facelift with home-made whipped cream. It's way better than store-bought, and it's quick and easy to make. The secret to making great whipped cream is to use a touch of vanilla extract. If you want it a bit sweeter, then whisk the cream with 1 tablespoon of sugar.*

Timesaving Tip: The easiest way to clean a whisk is to whisk it in a bowl of soapy water in the sink.

½ cup heavy cream
Dash vanilla extract
1 pint mixed fresh berries
4 mint leaves, for garnish

1. Place the heavy cream in a small bowl, and place the bowl inside of another larger bowl filled with ice.

2. Using a whisk, beat the cream until it thickens; the cream should just curl over softly when the whisk is held upright.

3. Whisk in the vanilla extract. Divide the berries into 4 bowls. Top the berries with the whipped cream and garnish with the mint leaves.

PER SERVING   CALORIES: 92   FAT: 6 G   TOTAL CARBOHYDRATES: 9 G
DIETARY FIBER: 3 G   SUGARS: 5 G   PROTEIN: 1 G

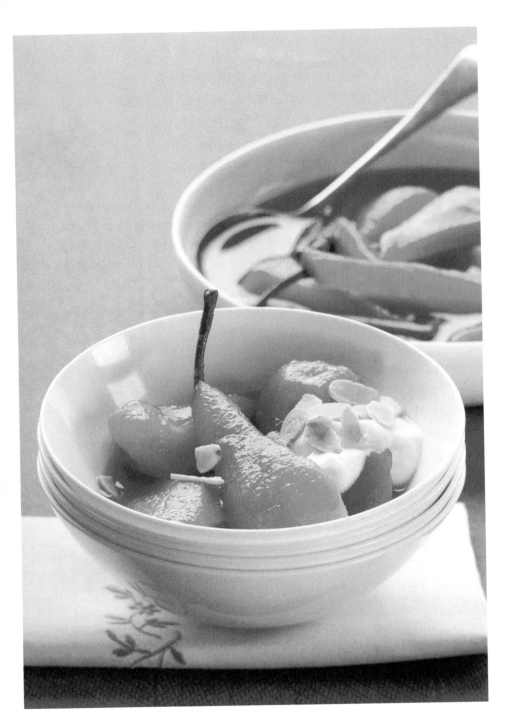

RED WINE–POACHED PEARS
WITH CRÈME FRAÎCHE

Nut-Free | Vegetarian

PREP TIME: 5 MINUTES ▲ COOK TIME: 30 MINUTES

SERVES 4   *Poaching pears is a simple way to create an elegant dessert. The technique of poaching involves immersing the pears partially in a liquid, such as wine, brandy, or even pear liqueur, and simmering them gently on the stovetop until they turn soft. The creamy sweetness of Bosc pears turns nice and mellow as they poach in the red wine, taking on the flavors of the wine in equal measure. It's probably wise to choose a bottle you would drink anyway, as the flavors will be concentrated.*

Timesaving Tip: A melon baller makes quick work of kitchen tasks like coring apples and pears. Cut the fruit in half, and use the melon baller to scoop out the center containing the seeds.

4 firm-ripe Bosc pears, peeled, halved, and seeded

3 cups red wine

¼ cup honey

1 cinnamon stick

3 cloves

Peel of 1 orange

¼ cup crème fraîche

2 tablespoons toasted sliced almonds, for garnish (optional)

1. Place the pears in a single layer in a wide skillet, and add the wine, honey, cinnamon stick, cloves, and orange peel.

2. Bring to a simmer, and cook for about 15 minutes per side, or until the pears are easily pierced with the tip of a knife.

3. Remove the pears from the poaching liquid, and serve with a dollop of crème fraîche on top. Garnish with the almonds (if using).

PER SERVING   CALORIES: 343   FAT: 1 G   TOTAL CARBOHYDRATES: 57 G
DIETARY FIBER: 8 G   SUGARS: 39 G   PROTEIN: 1 G

WHITE PEACH AND
BASIL GRANITA

Dairy-Free I Nut-Free I Paleo-Friendly I Vegetarian

PREP TIME: 10 MINUTES (PLUS FREEZING TIME)

SERVES 6   *A granita is similar to sorbet, but it is made with less sugar and has a grainier texture. Here, white peach and basil are the flavoring elements for the granita, and they are a great combination.*

Timesaving Tip: To make uniform pieces of basil, stack the basil leaves on top of one another and slice into them as you hold them in place.

1 cup hot water

¾ cup honey

3 cups finely diced white peaches

2 tablespoons finely chopped basil, for garnish

1. In a bowl, stir together the water and honey until they form a solution.

2. Combine the mixture with the white peaches in a blender, and process until smooth.

3. Strain into a shallow pan, and place in the freezer for 2 hours, scraping with a fork every half hour or so.

4. Scoop into bowls and garnish with basil to serve.

PER SERVING   CALORIES: 162   FAT: 0 G   TOTAL CARBOHYDRATES: 43 G
DIETARY FIBER: 1 G   SUGARS: 42 G   PROTEIN: 1 G

MULLED WINE WITH CINNAMON, CITRUS, AND CLOVE

Dairy-Free | Nut-Free | Paleo-Friendly | Vegan

PREP TIME: 5 MINUTES ⚊ COOK TIME: 15 MINUTES

SERVES 4   *On a chilly night, a cup of mulled wine makes a perfect companion. Its pleasant aroma comes from warm winter spices and refreshing citrus. For interesting variations, try changing the spice mix: star anise, juniper, and allspice are particularly nice.*

1 (750-mL) bottle red wine

1 cinnamon stick

3 whole cloves

Peel of 1 orange

Peel of 2 lemons

1. Into a large pot, pour the wine and add the cinnamon stick, cloves, and orange and lemon peels.

2. Bring to a boil, then simmer for 10 minutes.

3. Strain or ladle into heatproof cups.

PER SERVING   CALORIES: 133   FAT: 0 G   TOTAL CARBOHYDRATES: 8 G
DIETARY FIBER: 1 G   SUGARS: 2 G   PROTEIN: 0 G

Sauces, Dressings, and Condiments

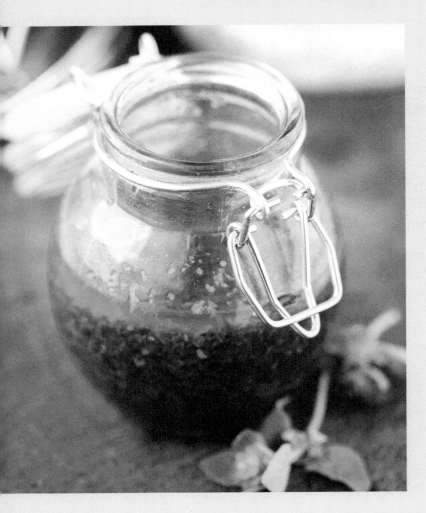

EASY PICO DE GALLO

Dairy-Free | Nut-Free | Paleo-Friendly | Vegan

PREP TIME: 10 MINUTES

SERVES 4 *Homemade pico de gallo is a snap to make and is all simple prep and no cooking. Add more finely chopped jalapeño pepper to the mix if you want it hotter.*

Timesaving Tip: Dicing an onion, when you really think about it, can be tricky. The fastest way to do it is a three-step process. First, cut the onion in half. Slice perpendicular to the root end (making sure not to go all the way to the root end). Second, slice toward the root end parallel to the cutting board (again, not going all the way through). Third, slice parallel to the root end to make an even dice.

2 pints cherry tomatoes, finely diced

½ red onion, finely diced

Juice of 1 lime

¼ cup finely chopped fresh cilantro leaves and stems

1 jalapeño pepper, seeded, stemmed, and finely diced (optional)

Sea salt

Freshly ground black pepper

1. In a medium bowl, mix together the tomatoes, onion, lime juice, cilantro, and jalapeño (if using).

2. Season with salt and pepper, and stir.

3. Make the salsa up to a day ahead, and store covered in the refrigerator.

PER SERVING CALORIES: 39 FAT: 0 G TOTAL CARBOHYDRATES: 9 G
DIETARY FIBER: 3 G SUGARS: 5 G PROTEIN: 2 G

ROMESCO

Dairy-Free | Paleo-Friendly | Vegan

PREP TIME: 10 MINUTES

SERVES 8   *Most romesco sauces are made with a mixture of tomatoes, roasted red peppers, toasted almonds and hazelnuts, red-wine or sherry vinegar, garlic, paprika, extra-virgin olive oil, and day-old bread. But it's just as good without the bread.*

Timesaving Tip: Make one recipe of the Romesco to use for all the other romesco-based dishes in this book. It can be kept in the refrigerator for up to 1 week.

- **3 roasted red peppers**
- **1 cup chopped tomatoes**
- **2 tablespoons sherry vinegar**
- **½ cup whole almonds, toasted**
- **½ cup hazelnuts, toasted**
- **2 garlic cloves, peeled**
- **½ teaspoon paprika**
- **½ cup extra-virgin olive oil**
- **Sea salt**
- **Freshly ground black pepper**

1. In the bowl of a food processor, place the red peppers, tomatoes, vinegar, almonds, hazelnuts, garlic, and paprika. Pulse until chopped.

2. With the machine running, slowly add in the oil until the sauce is smooth.

3. Season with salt and pepper.

4. The sauce can be made a day ahead and stored covered in the refrigerator.

PER SERVING   CALORIES: 184   FAT: 19 G   TOTAL CARBOHYDRATES: 5 G
DIETARY FIBER: 2 G   SUGARS: 2 G   PROTEIN: 2 G

QUICK MARINARA SAUCE

Dairy-Free I Nut-Free I Paleo-Friendly I Vegan

PREP TIME: 5 MINUTES ▲ COOK TIME: 10 MINUTES

SERVES 4   *This marinara sauce uses canned whole peeled tomatoes. Why not crushed? Crushed tomatoes are often made from tomatoes that are considered "seconds." They're perfectly safe for consumption but might not have the freshest flavor. Use a high-quality brand such as Muir Glen, or, if you can find them, true San Marzano tomatoes imported from Italy (not the San Marzano brand, which uses tomatoes that are grown in California and are not actually of the San Marzano variety).*

Timesaving Tip: If you prefer a thicker sauce, add a tablespoon of tomato paste with the garlic in step 2.

- 1 tablespoon extra-virgin olive oil
- 3 garlic cloves, chopped
- 1 (28-ounce) can whole peeled tomatoes
- Sea salt
- Freshly ground black pepper
- 1 cup torn basil leaves

1. In a medium pot, heat the oil over medium heat.

2. Add the garlic, and cook for 1 minute, or until golden.

3. Meanwhile, place the tomatoes in the bowl of a food processor, and process until smooth.

4. Pour the tomatoes into the pot, season with salt and pepper, increase the heat to high, and bring to a simmer. Simmer for 5 minutes, stirring, or until thickened slightly. Stir in the basil.

5. This sauce can be made one day ahead and stored in the refrigerator.

PER SERVING   CALORIES: 72   FAT: 4 G   TOTAL CARBOHYDRATES: 8 G
DIETARY FIBER: 2 G   SUGARS: 5 G   PROTEIN: 2 G

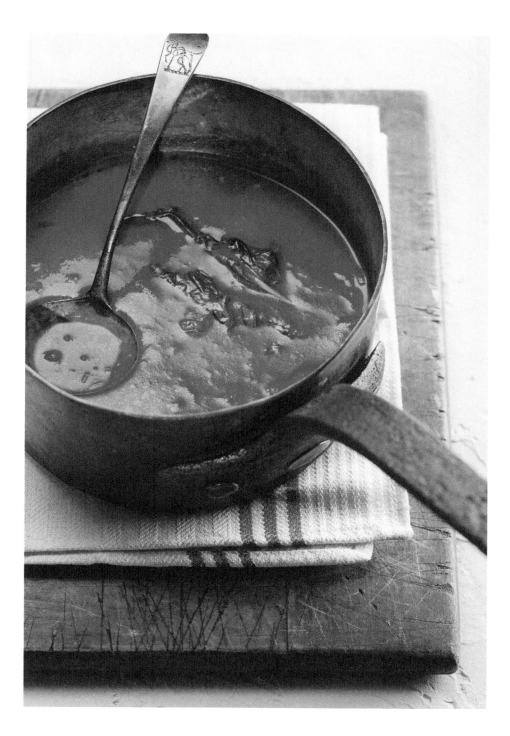

SIMPLE BASIL PESTO

Vegetarian

PREP TIME: 5 MINUTES

SERVES 8   *Pesto is so simple and quick to make at home. Basil pesto hails from the region of Liguria, located in the northwest of Italy. Liguria is also where pine nuts are grown, an ingredient that, depending on which Italian grandmother you ask, is either an essential or blasphemous ingredient in basil pesto. Thus, not wanting to anger anyone's grandmother, the pine nuts have been made optional in this recipe. Pine nuts can be rather expensive, so if you're looking to add nutty flavor to your pesto without breaking the bank, opt for almonds or walnuts instead.*

Diet Variation: To make this recipe dairy-free, omit the Parmesan.

1 bunch fresh basil leaves

½ cup grated Parmesan

¼ cup pine nuts, toasted (optional)

1 cup extra-virgin olive oil

Sea salt

Freshly ground black pepper

1. In the bowl of a food processor, put the basil leaves, Parmesan, and pine nuts and pulse until chopped.

2. With the machine running, slowly pour in the oil until the pesto becomes a thick purée.

3. Season with salt and pepper.

4. The pesto can be stored in the freezer for up to 3 months.

PER SERVING   CALORIES: 265   FAT: 29 G   TOTAL CARBOHYDRATES: 1 G
DIETARY FIBER: 0 G   SUGARS: 0 G   PROTEIN: 3 G

ARUGULA-WALNUT PESTO

Vegetarian

PREP TIME: 5 MINUTES

SERVES 8   *By swapping out the usual basil for arugula, and the usual pine nuts for walnuts, you get an interesting twist on the popular condiment. The spicy, peppery flavor of the arugula is complemented by the richness and slight bitterness of toasted walnuts. Use this pesto in much the same way as you would regular pesto. Pair with your favorite vegetable side dishes, grilled meats and poultry, and assertively flavored seafood.*

Diet Variation: To make this recipe dairy-free, omit the pecorino.

    2½ ounces baby arugula
    ¼ cup grated pecorino
    1 cup walnuts, toasted
    1 cup extra-virgin olive oil
    Sea salt
    Freshly ground black pepper

1. In the bowl of a food processor, put the arugula, pecorino, and walnuts and pulse until chopped.

2. With the machine running, slowly stream in the oil until combined.

3. Season with salt and pepper.

4. The pesto can be stored in the freezer for up to 3 months.

PER SERVING   CALORIES: 315   FAT: 35 G   TOTAL CARBOHYDRATES: 2 G
DIETARY FIBER: 1 G   SUGARS: 0 G   PROTEIN: 4 G

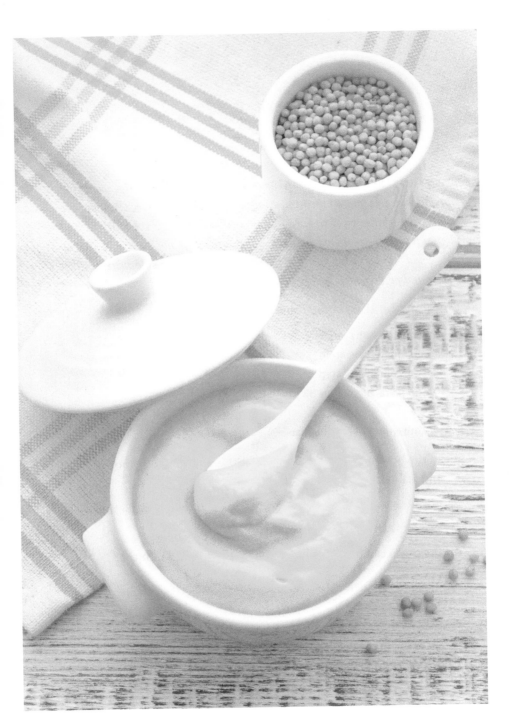

HOMEMADE MUSTARD

Dairy-Free | Nut-Free | Paleo-Friendly | Vegan

PREP TIME: 5 MINUTES (PLUS SOAKING TIME)

SERVES 20   *Once you make a batch of mustard, store-bought will never seem quite as good (or economical). Mustard seeds come in three main varieties: white, black, and brown. Experiment with different combinations to create your own house blend.*

- 1 cup whole mustard seeds
- 2 cups water
- 2 tablespoons distilled white vinegar

1. In a small bowl, soak the mustard seeds in the water until plump, about 8 hours or overnight.

2. Drain the seeds through a fine-mesh sieve. Put the seeds in the bowl of a food processor, add the vinegar, and process until it reaches the desired consistency—it should be fairly thick but spreadable.

3. Store covered in the refrigerator for up to 6 months.

PER SERVING   CALORIES: 37   FAT: 2 G   TOTAL CARBOHYDRATES: 3 G
DIETARY FIBER: 1 G   SUGARS: 1 G   PROTEIN: 2 G

TZATZIKI

Nut-Free | Vegetarian

PREP TIME: 10 MINUTES

SERVES 4   *Tzatziki, a Greek sauce made with yogurt, garlic, and cucumber, often accompanies gyros, a pita sandwich filled with grilled lamb, pork, or chicken and topped with lettuce and tomatoes. Tzatziki goes with just about any grilled meat dish and vegetables.*

Ingredient Tip: When buying garlic, look for firm, bright white heads free from blemishes. The cloves should be tightly bunched together.

- 1 (6-ounce) container nonfat plain Greek yogurt
- 6 garlic cloves, finely chopped
- ¼ cup finely diced cucumber
- ¼ cup finely diced red onion
- 1 teaspoon red wine vinegar
- ¼ cup water
- Sea salt

In a small bowl, stir together the yogurt, garlic, cucumber, onion, vinegar, and water until smooth. Season with salt. Store covered in the refrigerator for up to 1 week.

PER SERVING   CALORIES: 33   FAT: 0 G   TOTAL CARBOHYDRATES: 6 G
DIETARY FIBER: 1 G   SUGARS: 3 G   PROTEIN: 3 G

HOLLANDAISE SAUCE

Nut-Free

PREP TIME: 5 MINUTES ▲ COOK TIME: 10 MINUTES

SERVES 8 *With a little practice, you'll be whipping up hollandaise whenever you want with ease. For a variation, add a dash of cayenne pepper just before serving.*

This recipe makes use of ghee, or clarified butter. Many supermarkets now carry it, but if you can't find it, it's simple enough to make from unsalted regular butter. Simply melt the butter in a pan over low heat until the foam subsides and the solids begin to separate from the liquid. Skim out the solids using a spoon and use what is left behind.

Cooking Tip: If your hollandaise sauce curdles or breaks, incorporate the broken sauce into a new batch. At the step where you would add clarified butter, add the broken batch of sauce instead.

2 egg yolks

2 tablespoons water

7 ounces ghee, melted

Juice of ½ lemon

Sea salt

Cayenne pepper

1. In a medium pot, bring 1 inch of water to a simmer. Place a metal mixing bowl snugly over the top.

2. Crack the eggs into the bowl, add the water, and whisk continuously for about 4 minutes, or until the consistency resembles watery whipped cream. Lift the bowl periodically to check on the water and reduce the heat as necessary to maintain a steady simmer, or the eggs may scramble.

3. Add the ghee in a slow, steady stream while whisking until the sauce combines. »

4. Remove from the heat, and add the lemon juice and season with salt and cayenne pepper just before serving.

5. The sauce can be made up to 1 hour ahead of serving and kept at room temperature.

PER SERVING   CALORIES: 232   FAT: 26 G   TOTAL CARBOHYDRATES: 1 G
DIETARY FIBER: 0 G   SUGARS: 0 G   PROTEIN: 1 G

GARLIC AÏOLI

Dairy-Free | Nut-Free | Paleo-Friendly | Vegetarian

PREP TIME: 5 MINUTES

SERVES 16   *Aïoli is homemade mayonnaise that has an edgy flavor from a bit of raw garlic. It's good on anything you'd put regular mayonnaise on, including your favorite burgers, sandwiches, and coleslaw.*

- 1 egg
- 2 cups regular olive oil
- 1 garlic clove
- 1 tablespoon freshly squeezed lemon juice
- Sea salt
- Freshly ground black pepper

1. Place the egg in the bowl of a food processor.

2. With the machine running, slowly stream in the oil until thickened.

3. Add the garlic and lemon juice, season with salt and pepper, and process until the garlic is thoroughly incorporated.

4. Store covered in the refrigerator for up to 1 week.

PER SERVING   CALORIES: 220   FAT: 26 G   TOTAL CARBOHYDRATES: 0 G
DIETARY FIBER: 0 G   SUGARS: 0 G   PROTEIN: 0 G

CHIMICHURRI

Dairy-Free | Nut-Free | Paleo-Friendly | Vegan

PREP TIME: 5 MINUTES

SERVES 8   *This tangy, garlicky Argentinean condiment is the perfect match for a well-marbled steak, but it's also ideal with grilled fish and chicken. If you don't like cilantro, omit it and use more parsley.*

Ingredient Tip: This recipe makes use of both flat-leaf parsley and cilantro. While they may look alike and smell very different, you can also tell them apart visually when the herbs are fresh. Fresh cilantro has softer, brighter-looking leaves than flat-leaf parsley.

   3 cups chopped fresh flat-leaf parsley

   1 cup chopped fresh cilantro leaves and stems

   2 teaspoons red pepper flakes

   1 garlic clove

   3 tablespoons red-wine vinegar

   ½ cup extra-virgin olive oil

   Sea salt

   Freshly ground black pepper

1. In the bowl of a food processor, place the parsley, cilantro, red pepper flakes, garlic, and vinegar. Pulse until chopped.

2. With the machine running, add the oil and process until the sauce is smooth.

3. Season with salt and pepper, and pulse to combine.

4. The Chimichurri can be stored in the freezer for up to 3 months.

PER SERVING   CALORIES: 120   FAT: 13 G   TOTAL CARBOHYDRATES: 2 G
DIETARY FIBER: 1 G   SUGARS: 0 G   PROTEIN: 1 G

CHARMOULA

Dairy-Free | Nut-Free | Paleo-Friendly | Vegan

PREP TIME: 10 MINUTES

SERVES 8   *Charmoula is typically served with fish or seafood since its vibrant flavor contrasts wonderfully with the flavors of the sea. For an interesting variation, try adding dried red chiles.*

Ingredient Tip: Reserve extra-virgin olive oil for dressings and for use as a finishing oil. If you must absolutely cook with it, do not exceed temperatures of 350°F in the oven, or medium heat on the stove. High temperatures cause extra-virgin olive oil to lose its flavor. For high-heat applications, use pure, light, or extra-light olive oil.

3 cups chopped fresh cilantro

½ teaspoon ground cumin

½ teaspoon paprika

1 garlic clove

Juice of ½ lemon

½ cup extra-virgin olive oil

Sea salt

Freshly ground black pepper

1. In the bowl of a food processor, place the cilantro, cumin, paprika, garlic, and lemon juice. Pulse until chopped.

2. With the machine running, add the oil until the sauce is smooth.

3. Season with salt and pepper, and pulse to combine.

4. The Charmoula can be stored in the freezer for up to 3 months.

PER SERVING   CALORIES: 112   FAT: 13 G   TOTAL CARBOHYDRATES: 1 G
DIETARY FIBER: 0 G   SUGARS: 0 G   PROTEIN: 0 G

OLIVE TAPENADE

Dairy-Free | Nut-Free | Paleo-Friendly

PREP TIME: 5 MINUTES ⏣ COOK TIME: 2 MINUTES

SERVES 6   *Olive Tapenade is a condiment made with black olives, olive oil, garlic, anchovies, capers, and lemon juice. It originates from Provence, a region in the south of France.*

Ingredient Variation: Add some green olives, such as picholines, in the mix for a brinier flavor.

4 tablespoons extra-virgin olive oil, divided

2 anchovy fillets

2 garlic cloves, chopped

1 cup pitted black olives, such as Gaeta or Kalamata, drained and rinsed

1 tablespoon capers, drained and rinsed

1 teaspoon red pepper flakes

Juice of ½ lemon

Sea salt

Freshly ground black pepper

1. In a small skillet, heat 1 tablespoon of the oil together with the anchovies and garlic over medium-low heat for about 1 to 2 minutes, just until they start to sizzle and the oil is warmed.

2. Place the olives, capers, red pepper flakes, and lemon juice in the bowl of a food processor, and with the machine running, slowly add the remaining 3 tablespoons of oil. Add the anchovies and garlic to the mixture.

3. Season with salt and pepper.

4. Store covered for up to 1 week.

PER SERVING   CALORIES: 105   FAT: 11 G   TOTAL CARBOHYDRATES: 2 G
DIETARY FIBER: 1 G   SUGARS: 0 G   PROTEIN: 1 G

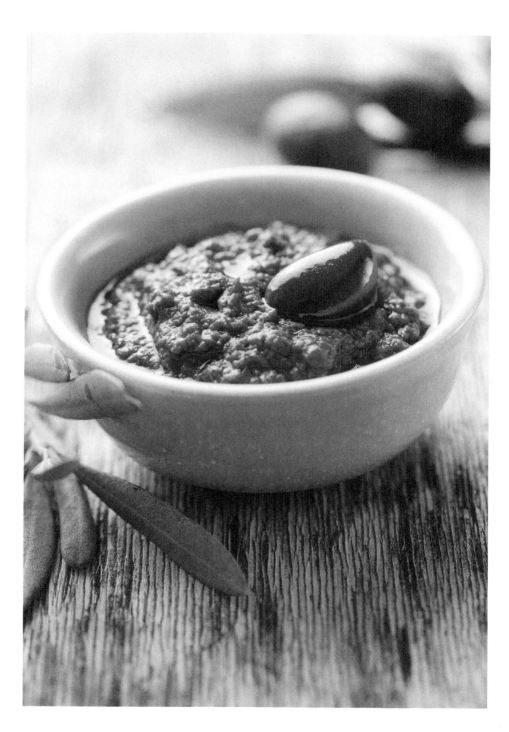

LEMON VINAIGRETTE

Dairy-Free | Nut-Free | Paleo-Friendly | Vegan

PREP TIME: 5 MINUTES

SERVES 8   *This dressing is used frequently with the recipes in this book. Use it as a template for making other salad dressings. The classic ratio for oil to acid is 3:1, but if you like your dressing a bit more tangy, use less oil. This versatile dressing can be used on your favorite salad recipes, but it's also great with seafood and chicken.*

Ingredient Tip: Purchase extra-virgin olive oil that comes in dark bottles. The dark bottles help protect the antioxidant compounds in the oil which also carry its flavor and aroma. Exposure to light causes these compounds to degrade more quickly.

2 garlic cloves, grated
¼ cup freshly squeezed lemon juice
Sea salt
Freshly ground black pepper
¾ cup extra-virgin olive oil

1. In a medium bowl, place the garlic in the lemon juice. Season with salt and pepper.

2. While whisking, slowly add the oil until the dressing is thick and combined.

3. Make the dressing up to a day ahead, and store covered in the refrigerator. Let it come to room temperature before using, and whisk to combine again.

PER SERVING   CALORIES: 165   FAT: 19 G   TOTAL CARBOHYDRATES: 0 G
DIETARY FIBER: 0 G   SUGARS: 0 G   PROTEIN: 0 G

MUSTARD VINAIGRETTE

Dairy-Free | Nut-Free | Paleo-Friendly | Vegan

PREP TIME: 5 MINUTES

SERVES 8   *It's amazing how the addition of just one ingredient can sometimes transform the entire flavor of the recipe. Such is the case with this Mustard Vinaigrette, which begins much like the Lemon Vinaigrette (page 286). The mustard acts both as a flavoring agent and an emulsifier, which helps keep the dressing from separating for longer periods of time.*

2 garlic cloves, grated

¼ cup freshly squeezed lemon juice

2 tablespoons mustard

Sea salt

Freshly ground black pepper

¾ cup extra-virgin olive oil

1. In a medium bowl, place the garlic in the lemon juice and mustard. Season with salt and pepper.

2. While whisking, slowly stream in the olive oil until combined.

3. Make the dressing up to a day ahead, and store covered in the refrigerator. Let it come to room temperature before using, and whisk to combine again if necessary.

PER SERVING   CALORIES: 178   FAT: 20 G   TOTAL CARBOHYDRATES: 1 G
DIETARY FIBER: 0 G   SUGARS: 0 G   PROTEIN: 1 G

GREEK YOGURT–DILL DRESSING

Nut-Free | Vegetarian

PREP TIME: 5 MINUTES

SERVES 6   *Fans of creamy dressings often have trouble switching to lighter vinaigrettes. Some resort to using low-fat, store-bought mayonnaise, which often has more sugar and salt than its full-fat counterparts (the loss of flavor has to be compensated for somehow, right?). Here's a better solution: nonfat Greek yogurt. It transforms the classic Lemon Vinaigrette (page 286) into a creamy yet light dressing that's fit for sturdier greens like kale and hearty salad classics like potato salad.*

- **6 tablespoons extra-virgin olive oil**
- **2 tablespoons freshly squeezed lemon juice**
- **1 (6-ounce) container nonfat Greek yogurt**
- **¼ cup chopped fresh dill**
- **Sea salt**
- **Freshly ground black pepper**

1. In a medium bowl, slowly whisk the oil into the lemon juice until combined, then whisk in the Greek yogurt.

2. Add the chopped dill, and season with salt and pepper.

3. Make the dressing up to a day ahead, and store covered in the refrigerator. Let it come to room temperature before using, and whisk to combine again.

PER SERVING   CALORIES: 143   FAT: 14 G   TOTAL CARBOHYDRATES: 2 G
DIETARY FIBER: 0 G   SUGARS: 1 G   PROTEIN: 3 G

BUTTERMILK DRESSING

Nut-Free | Vegetarian

PREP TIME: 5 MINUTES

SERVES 8   *Looking for the perfect dressing for your pan-fried fish, bold salad, or refreshing slaw? Try this Buttermilk Dressing, which is lighter than many of the typical buttermilk dressing recipes. This one is more of a vinaigrette since it incorporates vinegar and olive oil, and it lends itself to dishes that require a creamy dressing that's not too heavy.*

Ingredient Variation: Add a teaspoon or two of finely chopped garlic to add a different spin on the flavor.

- ¼ cup regular olive oil
- ¼ cup buttermilk
- 2 tablespoons apple cider vinegar
- Sea salt
- Freshly ground black pepper

1. In a medium bowl, whisk the oil into the buttermilk and vinegar.

2. Season with salt and pepper.

3. Make the dressing up to a day ahead, and store covered in the refrigerator. Let it come to room temperature before using, and whisk to combine again if necessary.

PER SERVING CALORIES: 58 FAT: 6 G   TOTAL CARBOHYDRATES: 0 G
DIETARY FIBER: 0 G SUGARS: 0 G PROTEIN: 0 G

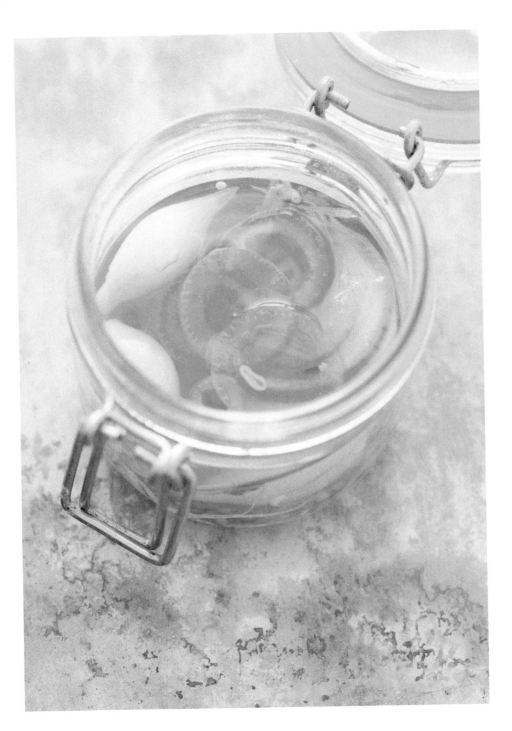

PICKLED ONIONS

Dairy-Free | Nut-Free | Paleo-Friendly | Vegetarian

PREP TIME: 20 MINUTES ▲ COOK TIME: 5 MINUTES

SERVES 4   *Chefs and home cooks are pickling everything from beets and cauliflower to garlic and onions. They're not just limiting themselves to vegetables either: Pickled watermelon rinds, cherries, and even eggs are found on today's tables. But pickling most vegetables takes a fair amount of time and requires sterilizing jars, a cumbersome process. On the short list, though: onions. Try serving them with your favorite salads, vegetable sides, and grilled meats.*

Cooking Tip: When slicing an onion, you can make thinner slices more easily if you use your free hand to guide the knife. Curl up the fingers of your free hand into a "C" with your thumb tucked safely behind your other fingers. Place those fingers at the edge of the next slice, and move them down the onion as you slice. You should feel the flat side of the blade with each slice.

- 2 tablespoons honey
- 2 teaspoons sea salt
- 1 cup apple cider vinegar
- 1 red onion, sliced thinly

1. In a medium saucepan, bring the honey, salt, and vinegar to a boil over high heat, and cook until the salt is dissolved.

2. Add the onion, and submerge for about 20 minutes, or until it softens and changes color.

3. When the onion is ready to use, drain and let cool. Store covered in the refrigerator for up to 2 weeks, and drain before using.

PER SERVING   CALORIES: 56   FAT: 0 G   TOTAL CARBOHYDRATES: 12 G
DIETARY FIBER: 1 G   SUGARS: 10 G   PROTEIN: 0 G

HOMEMADE PEANUT SAUCE

Dairy-Free | Vegetarian

PREP TIME: 5 MINUTES

SERVES 8   *Peanut sauce is an essential condiment in various Southeast Asian cuisines, including Thai, Malaysian, Vietnamese, and Indonesian. Most people will be familiar with it from chicken or beef satay skewers. All you need to make it is three ingredients: peanuts, honey, and water.*

1 cup unsalted peanuts
2 tablespoons honey
½ cup water

1. In the bowl of a food processor, put the peanuts and honey and pulse until combined.

2. With the machine running, gradually add the water until the sauce is slightly grainy while still runny. It should not turn creamy like peanut butter; there should still be some texture.

3. Store any leftover sauce, covered, in the refrigerator for up to 1 week.

PER SERVING   CALORIES: 119   FAT: 9 G   TOTAL CARBOHYDRATES: 7 G
DIETARY FIBER: 2 G   SUGARS: 5 G   PROTEIN: 5 G

CHOCOLATE SAUCE

Nut-Free | Vegetarian

SERVES 16   *Use this intensely flavored Chocolate Sauce for everything from topping sundaes and banana splits to flavoring your favorite milkshakes. Use the highest quality chocolate you can find; it's best to pick the chocolate with the fewest number of ingredients, a sign that usually indicates less processing was involved. For an even more intense flavor, use bittersweet chocolate.*

- 1 pound semisweet chocolate chips
- ¼ cup milk
- 2 tablespoons honey

1. Bring 1 inch of water to a simmer in a medium pot, and place a bowl snugly over the top.
2. Add the chocolate and melt, stirring occasionally with a spatula.
3. Stir in the milk and honey.
4. Store covered in the refrigerator for up to 1 week.

PER SERVING   CALORIES: 150   FAT: 8 G   TOTAL CARBOHYDRATES: 20 G
DIETARY FIBER: 2 G   SUGARS: 16 G   PROTEIN: 0 G

STRAWBERRY COULIS

Dairy-Free | Nut-Free | Paleo-Friendly | Vegetarian

PREP TIME: 10 MINUTES ▲ COOK TIME: 10 MINUTES

SERVES 8   *Sometimes, store-bought strawberry sauce can be overly sweet. Strawberry Coulis can be thought of as a more refined version, made with fresh strawberries and lemon juice, and here, sweetened with honey. Serve with your favorite classics like sundaes, banana splits, and milkshakes.*

1 pound fresh strawberries, finely diced

½ cup honey

Juice of ½ lemon

1. Place the strawberries in a medium pot with the honey and lemon juice over low heat, and simmer until the strawberries are soft.

2. Transfer to a blender, and blend until smooth.

3. Store covered in the refrigerator for up to 1 week.

PER SERVING   CALORIES: 84   FAT: 0 G   TOTAL CARBOHYDRATES: 22 G
DIETARY FIBER: 1 G   SUGARS: 20 G   PROTEIN: 1 G

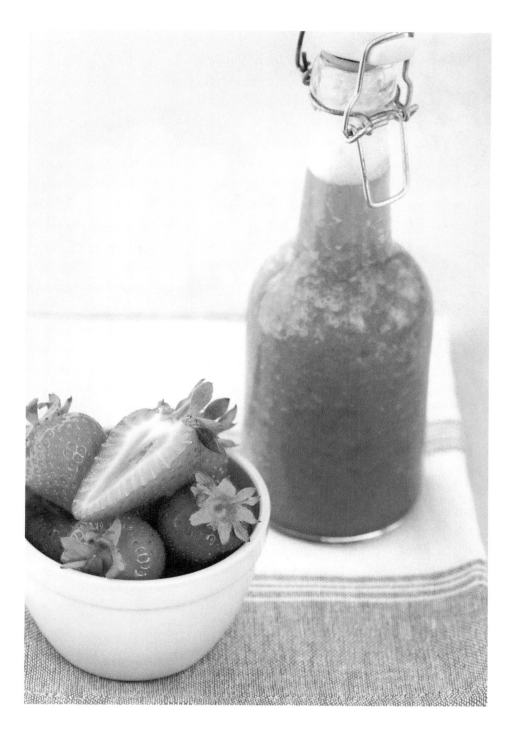

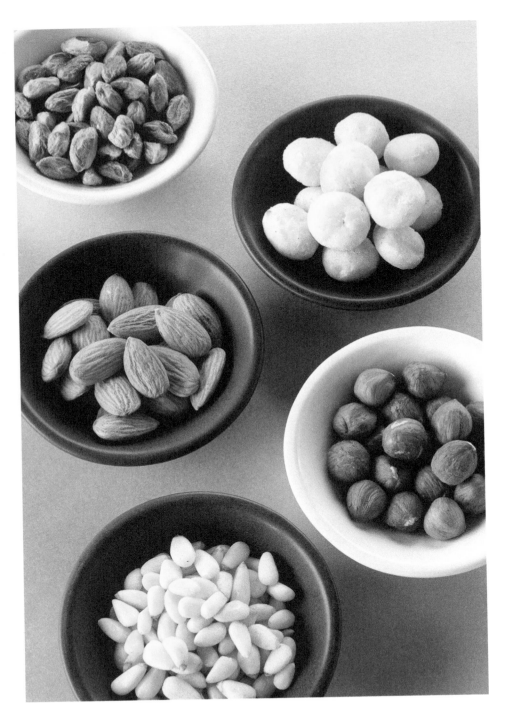

Appendix A 10 Tips for Eating Out

While ideally you would cook every meal you eat as part of your new grain-free lifestyle, that's just not realistic. Let's face it, at some point or another, you're going to end up eating in restaurants. Fortunately there are tips to help you navigate most restaurant menus with confidence. Here, experts weigh in with their advice on what to do when dining out.

1. **Don't leave things to chance.** Jennifer Knollenberg, nutritional analyst and recipe developer for Atkins Nutritionals, says, "Do not be afraid to ask what the ingredients are in a meal. Most restaurants are happy to accommodate changes. Be specific, ask what vegetables they are serving and ask to substitute those for the pasta, potatoes, or rice in a dish."

2. **Out of sight, out of mind.** She says, "If a meal comes with something tempting such as French fries, or dried cranberries on a salad, or a bun on a hamburger, request that it be removed from the table or prepared without it. A lot of us have the notion that we are wasting food or must clear our plates, so often removing them yourself doesn't remove the temptation to have just one or two (which leads to three or four or more) French fries."

3. **What about dessert?** Desserts are a land mine of grains and grain products. If everyone at your table is ordering dessert, Knollenberg advises that you order your favorite beverage—coffee, tea, or perhaps a glass of wine—so you don't feel left out. Many restaurants also offer a fruit and cheese plate as an option.

4. **Ask about gluten-free menus.** Many chain restaurants and independent establishments now offer gluten-free menus. While not grain-free, they are often a good place to start, since some of the options may be grain-free.

5. **Avoid soy sauce.** There are many hidden sources of wheat, but this is one of the most common (and still relatively unknown sources) when dining out.

6. **Help the staff take you seriously.** William Davis, MD, author of *Wheat Belly*, knows it can be difficult sometimes to capture the attention of people who aren't following a grain-free diet. If, for example, you're at a restaurant and you're determined to stay grain-free, tell the staff that you have a food allergy. It's a bit extreme, perhaps, but it's simple and effective.

7. **What about traveling?** Dining options at airports can be relatively narrow, and anyone who follows a restricted diet (not just grain-free) can run into trouble trying to find something to eat. That's why it's probably a good idea to plan in advance and bring some snacks with you from home. Some good options include nuts and seeds, nut butters with chopped vegetables for dipping, homemade dips like hummus and guacamole, and salads that don't have too many leafy greens (which can turn soggy).

8. **Keep it simple.** David Perlmutter, MD, author of *Grain Brain*, cautions against "elaborate dishes that contain multiple ingredients." In other words, stick to what you know, and you'll know what you're getting. For example, ask for your fish or chicken grilled without any sauce.

9. **Be realistic.** Dr. Perlmutter likes to stick to the 80/20 rule, but aims for 90/10. What does that mean? Simply put, the 80/20 rule as it applies to the grain-free diet would be, "Eat grain-free 80 percent of the time, and indulge 20 percent of the time." But human nature being the way it is, it's probably a good idea to aim a little higher so that you're not disappointed when you fall short. Aim for 90/10, and you'll naturally end up at 80/20. The ideal grain-free dieter would hit 100 percent all the time, but for most people, that's just not realistic.

10. **Accept the consequences.** If you find yourself in a situation where only foods with grains are served, make your peace with it. Dr. Perlmutter says, "Be willing to accept those consequences if you cannot say no."

Appendix B Measurement Conversions

Volume Equivalents (Liquid)

US STANDARD (OUNCES)	US STANDARD	METRIC (APPROX-IMATE)
2 tablespoons	1 fl. oz.	30 mL
¼ cup	2 fl. oz.	60 mL
½ cup	4 fl. oz.	120 mL
1 cup	8 fl. oz.	240 mL
1½ cups	12 fl. oz.	355 mL
2 cups or 1 pint	16 fl. oz.	475 mL
4 cups or 1 quart	32 fl. oz.	1 L
1 gallon	128 fl. oz.	4 L

Oven Temperatures

FAHRENHEIT (F)	CELSIUS (C) (APPROXIMATE)
250	120
300	150
325	165
350	180
375	190
400	200
425	220
450	230

Volume Equivalents (Dry)

US STANDARD	METRIC (APPROXIMATE)
⅛ teaspoon	.5 mL
¼ teaspoon	1 mL
½ teaspoon	2 mL
¾ teaspoon	4 mL
1 teaspoon	5 mL
1 tablespoon	15 mL
¼ cup	59 mL
⅓ cup	79 mL
½ cup	118 mL
⅔ cup	156 mL
¾ cup	177 mL
1 cup	235 mL
2 cups or 1 pint	475 mL
3 cups	700 mL
4 cups or 1 quart	1 L
½ gallon	2 L
1 gallon	4 L

Weight Equivalents

US STANDARD	METRIC (APPROXIMATE)
½ ounce	15 g
1 ounce	30 g
2 ounces	60 g
4 ounces	115 g
8 ounces	225 g
12 ounces	340 g
16 ounces or 1 pound	455 g

Resources

BOOKS

Davis, William. *Wheat Belly: Lose the Wheat, Lose the Weight, and Find Your Path Back to Health*. New York: Rodale, 2011.

Perlmutter, David. *Grain Brain: The Surprising Truth about Wheat, Carbs, and Sugar—Your Brain's Silent Killers*. New York: Little, Brown and Company, 2013.

Walker, Danielle. *Against the Grain: Delectable Paleo Recipes to Eat Well & Feel Great*. Las Vegas: Victory Press Publishing Inc., 2013.

WEBSITES

Against All Grain
http://againstallgrain.com/

Gluten Free Guide's Chain Restaurant Gluten Free Menu List
http://glutenfreeguidehq.com/chain-restaurants/

Paleo Primal Post
http://paleoprimalpost.com

Red Boat Fish Sauce
www.redboatfishsauce.com

USDA National Nutrient Database
http://ndb.nal.usda.gov/ndb/foods

US Wellness Meats
www.uswellnessmeats.com

References

American Diabetes Association. "Statistics about Diabetes." Accessed June 9, 2014. www.diabetes.org/diabetes-basics/statistics/.

Celiac Disease Foundation. "What is Celiac Disease?" Accessed October 2, 2014. http://celiac.org/celiac-disease/what-is-celiac-disease/

Davis, William. *Wheat Belly: Lose the Wheat, Lose the Weight, and Find Your Path Back to Health.* New York: Rodale, 2011.

Gould, Lauren (personal trainer; health and nutrition coach, American Association of Drugless Practitioners), in discussion with Will Budiaman, June 2014.

Heimowitz, Colette (vice president of nutrition and education, Atkins Nutritionals Inc.), in discussion with Will Budiaman, June 2014.

Hyman, Mark. "Three Hidden Ways Wheat Makes You Fat." *Huffington Post.* Accessed May 6, 2014. www.huffingtonpost.com/dr-mark -hyman/wheat-gluten_b_1274872.html.

Juntunen KS, Niskanen LK, Liukkonen KH, Poutanen KS, Holst JJ, Mykkänen HM. "Postprandial Glucose, Insulin, and Incretin Responses to Grain Products in Healthy Subjects." *American Journal of Clinical Nutrition* 75, no. 2 (February 2002): 254–62. http://ajcn .nutrition.org/content/75/2/254.full.

Knollenberg, Jennifer (nutritional analyst and recipe developer, Atkins Nutritionals Inc.), in discussion with Will Budiaman, June 2014.

Parks, Elizabeth J, Mark K Hellerstein. "Carbohydrate-Induced Hypertriacylglycerolemia: Historical Perspective and Review of Biological Mechanisms." *American Journal of Clinical Nutrition* 71, no. 4 (February 2000): 12–23. http://ajcn.nutrition.org/content/71 /2/412.full.

Perlmutter, David. *Grain Brain: The Surprising Truth about Wheat, Carbs, and Sugar—Your Brain's Silent Killers.* New York: Little, Brown and Company, 2013.

Shepherd, Sue, and Peter Gibson. *The Complete Low-FODMAP Diet: A Revolutionary Plan for Managing IBS and Other Digestive Disorders.* New York: The Experiment, 2013.

Valpone, Amie (editor in chief, TheHealthyApple.com), in discussion with Will Budiaman, June 2014.

Webb, Robyn (food editor, *Diabetes Forecast* magazine), in discussion with Will Budiaman, June 2014.

Zioudrou, C., RA Streaty, WA Klee. "Opioid Peptides Derived from Food Proteins. The Exorphins." *Journal of Biological Chemistry*, April 10, 1979, 2446–49. www.jbc.org/content/254/7/2446.abstract.

Recipe Index

Index

F

Fats, increasing intake of healthy, 8

Feta cheese, 29
  Cherry Tomato Salad with Feta and Basil, 86
  Greek Salad with Lemon Vinaigrette, 85
  Grilled Chicken Cobb Salad with Smoked Bacon, 76–77
  Grilled Zucchini and Eggplant Salad with Feta and Red Onion, 153
  Peach, Feta, and Mint Caprese Salad, 138
  Vegetarian Stuffed Cabbage, 162–163

Fish and Seafood, 164–197
  Baby Shrimp Ceviche with Mango, Radish, and Red Onion, 97
  Baked Tilapia with Ginger and Scallions, 179
  Cioppino, 188–190
  Grilled Branzino with Easy Pico de Gallo, 183
  Grilled Salmon with Olive Tapenade, 185
  Marinated Barbecued Shrimp, 168
  Pan-Fried Trout with Black Peppercorn–Buttermilk Dressing, 177–178
  Pan-Roasted Salmon with Pickled Onions and Mustard Vinaigrette, 182
  Pan-Roasted Trout with Pesto, 195
  Pan-Seared Shrimp with Arugula-Walnut Pesto, 167
  Pan-Seared Tilapia with Olive Tapenade and Lemon Zest, 174
  Poached Fresh Cod with Grape Tomatoes, Capers, and Olives, 186–187
  Roasted Shrimp with Tzatziki, 170
  Seared Calamari with Lemon and Capers, 180
  Seared Scallops with Lemon-Herb Vinaigrette, 166
  Seared Scallops with Pickled Onions and Charmoula, 193
  Shrimp Fra Diavolo, 196–197
  Shrimp Scampi with Quinoa, 175–176
  South Indian–Style Fish Curry, 191–192
  Steamed Mussels with Parsley, Lemon, and Shallot, 173
  Thai Steamed Mussels with Ginger, Lemongrass, and Chiles, 171

Fish sauce, 29

Flan, 246

Fluffy Mashed Cauliflower with Thyme, 121

Food processors, 25

Food ruts, falling into, 16

French-Style Potato Salad with Dijon Vinaigrette, 92–93

French-Style Scrambled Eggs, 56

Fresh Artichoke-Lemon Dip, 111–112

Fresh Strawberry Yogurt Smoothie, 53

Fresh Summer Bean Salad, 104–105

Frittata with Tomato and Parmesan, 66

Fruits, dried, 26

G

Garlic
  Chicken Salad with Garlic Aïoli, 84
  Easy Roast Chicken with Rosemary and Garlic, 228
  Garlic Aïoli, 281
  Garlic Hummus with Tahini, 114
  Gribiche, 91
  Mexican Grilled Corn, 117

Ghee, 279
  Hollandaise Sauce, 279–280

Gluten-free bread, 27

Gluten-free diets, 18

Glycemic index, 2

Goat cheese
  Soft Scrambled Eggs with Goat Cheese and Chives, 57

Gould, Lauren, 6, 8

Grain Brain (Perlmutter), 1, 5, 298

Grain Brain diet, 3

Grain-free, culinary tips for cooking, 27

Grain-free and gluten-free cheat sheet, 19

Grain-free diets
  drinking alcohol on, 18
  great ingredients for, 28–29
  guidelines for, 6–9
  overview of, 3
  switching to, vii
  tips for following, 15–17

Grain-free lifestyle, gearing up for, 20–33

Grains
  breaking free from, 10–19
  defined, vii
  effects of eating, 1–2
  reasons hard to quit, 11–12

CPSIA information can be obtained at www.ICGtesting.com
Printed in the USA
BVOW11s0947111114

374544BV00001B/1/P